the hormone shift

the hormone shift

Balance Your Body and Thrive Through Midlife and Menopause

Tasneem Bhatia, MD

goop
PRESS

RODALE
NEW YORK

Library of Congress Cataloging-in-Publication Data
Names: Bhatia, Tasneem, author.
Title: The hormone shift / Tasneem Bhatia, MD
Description: New York : Goop Press, [2023] | Includes index.
Identifiers: LCCN 2023016675 (print) | LCCN 2023016676 (ebook) |
ISBN 9780593578698 (hardback) | ISBN 9780593578711 (trade paperback) |
ISBN 9780593578704 (epub)
Subjects: LCSH: Menopause—Alternative treatment. | Middle-aged women—
Health and hygiene. | Hormone therapy. | Hormones.
Classification: LCC RG186 .B525 2023 (print) | LCC RG186 (ebook) |
DDC 618.1/75—dc23/eng/20230710
LC record available at https://lccn.loc.gov/2023016675
LC ebook record available at https://lccn.loc.gov/2023016676

ISBN 978-0-593-57869-8
Ebook ISBN 978-0-593-57870-4

Printed in the United States of America

Book design by Andrea Lau
Jacket design by Irene Ng
Jacket illustration by Hanna Barczyk
Author photograph courtesy of the author

10 9 8 7 6 5 4 3 2 1

First Edition

contents

PART I

Dump the Baggage and Clear the Blockages

PART II

Superpowered: The EastWest Approach to Hormone Balance

PART III
Resetting Your Hormones

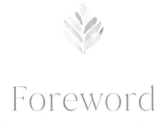

Foreword

I was talking to Dr. Taz a couple of years ago about turning fifty. She told me that she saw fifty as a culmination of the first part of our lives and an opportunity to reflect and decide how we want to live the next half. Taz described this chapter of our lives as the journey to becoming who you are—discovering your true soul, your essence, your purpose for being here.

Taz's work as an integrative practitioner and hormone expert is so brilliant because her approach embraces the idea that, as she says, we're rising into our power and into our truth. And at the same time, she deeply understands that we need different kinds of support to navigate these later phases of our life with vibrancy. Many of us struggle with hormonal changes leading up to and throughout perimenopause and menopause. There is no way to bypass this journey, but there are, thankfully, many things we can do to make it a smoother one.

In *The Hormone Shift*, Taz starts by helping you come to an understanding of how your hormones function and how to optimize them to help you feel your best. Her toolbox is wide and nuanced, but the levers she shows you how to pull are often blessedly simple. Sometimes, as she's seen again and again, just a couple of tweaks here and there really do make all the difference.

Thinking back to that conversation we had years ago, I remember Taz told me that she wouldn't accept the assumption that women are done at a certain age because she still has a lot to do. Since that conversation, I've entered my fifties—and there's still a lot I hope to do. And like Taz and her patients and my friends and so many women I know, we all want to feel vital while we're doing it—even when the "it" is accepting an invitation to soften and slow down a bit.

Taz and I both believe that we need to get rid of the idea that women expire at fifty (or forty, or sixty, or any age). And more so, we believe we need to embrace the new and exciting potential that exists within each of us in our later decades—a kind of power that most of us did not have access to in our younger years.

I'm so grateful that Taz has given us the gift of this book. It encompasses the kind of conversation so many of us have been eager and curious to have around hormones and aging and vitality. It outlines the information about our bodies that all women should have access to, long before they reach perimenopause—so that they can move through earlier hormonal changes with more ease and even look forward to, instead of dread, later ones.

Another wise woman, fifteen years ahead of me, told me that the final third of a woman's life is a time when she gives birth to herself—

when she finally mothers herself. *The Hormone Shift* is a beautiful guide to that worthy endeavor, a manual to help us understand how we can best care for, nourish, and show grace to ourselves. And it's also a bright reminder of the incredible impact that we can have on our own relationships and on the wider world when we do so.

—Gwyneth Paltrow, founder and CEO of goop

the hormone shift

introduction

The Stranger in the Mirror

Have you ever looked in the mirror and not recognized the person you see there? The woman staring back at you may feel unfamiliar, with a body that seems different from the one you know and love. Or, her skin may be duller, her hair may be thinning; there might be belly fat you've not seen before. Perhaps this view makes your mind feel clouded and your emotions volatile. Maybe you're feeling your energy is not as high as usual. Or, you can't remember the last time you slept through the night. All this leaves you wondering . . .

What the @#>! is going on here?

And then it hits you. . . . Ahhh—*I must be getting old.*

This is the biggest lie that's ever been told to women, and it took hundreds, maybe even thousands, of years to weave its components together. And today we still believe it.

I wish I could count the number of times these words (or a variation on them) have been said to me by the women I meet every day in my practice at CentreSpringMD, those in my community, and others in the audiences to whom I speak. I have heard those words over and over again during the last fifteen years of my practice. Whether the women are in their thirties or their fifties, they use the same line, the same language; it's almost as if they are watching me and waiting to see how long it will take for me to break and nod my head in agreement. We *must* be getting old, right? How else can we explain that stranger we see in the mirror—that image slowly morphing into an unrecognizable, duller version of our earlier selves? It's aging; it's normal. It's the settling into our mother's perimenopause and menopause, the time when our clothes just have to get bigger, our muscles are expected to disappear. Those abs, well, they're a thing of the past, right?

Wrong! That's the trap to be avoided.

We're up against almost 250 years—if not more—of conditioning when we try to fight this old narrative. But your mother's, grandmother's, and great-grandmother's perimenopause and menopause are not your story. Honestly, it should not have been theirs either. When the average woman's life span was sixty years, approaching the fifty-year mark with some trepidation was understandable. But when most of us are living past eighty, even ninety, fifty is not old.

For too long now, perimenopause and menopause have been relegated to the shadows. There's something about reaching this stage of life that has been seen as admitting defeat or achieving irrelevance. It doesn't help that the stereotypical hormonal symptoms are easy to mock—the butt of constant jokes in the media and even by loved ones. As a result, women have tried to hide those symptoms because they didn't want people to know they were now experiencing them. I think that, in their heads, women's acknowledgment of these symptoms was a confession that they, indeed, *might be old.*

Here's the truth: age really is a number. Our hormones shift throughout our lives, as they should, and how well we handle these shifts leads us to soul alignment. Many women today are not aware that there are myriad ways of navigating the hormone shifts—and that there are ways to work with your hormones to achieve balance and minimize those symptoms. That's true only if we understand that hormone shifts are transitions—transitions that come with a gift and a lesson that bring us closer to achieving our purpose. And who wants to keep that gift and lesson trapped or hidden?

While I see many women in my practice every day who have fallen into that old-age trap, an equal number are demanding a better way. And that's what I can offer them. With help, they emerge stronger, more confident, and healthier. They become their own advocates, and they are testimony to the simple fact that, as research is proving, age is just a number.

My Story

I'm so passionate about rewriting this centuries-old narrative because I've been there, too—been in what I call Hormone Hell, feeling like a shadow of myself. I know how that feeling can impact your entire life, including every decision you make. If I had stayed in that space, I surely would not have been vibrant enough to speak publicly, to run companies, or even to have nourishing relationships.

In 1997, I was twenty-eight years old, and I was your classic adrenaline junkie. After finishing my studies at the Medical College of Georgia, in Augusta, I took a job working in a busy hospital emergency room in Atlanta, managing injuries, infections, and full-out trauma, with an insane schedule that did not differentiate day from night. There was no "work–life balance"; it was all work, all the time. And that meant an even harder personal life. I was burning the candle at both ends and trying to hold it all together—or so I thought. And then the shit hit the fan.

Out of nowhere—or so it seemed—my hair was falling out. I'd packed on the pounds and my knees hurt. The endless cups of coffee couldn't help me beat the fatigue I felt every day.

What the **** was going on?!

I was the last person who would ever admit there was a problem (that would mean shame and guilt, on full display!). I was young, fresh out of school, with a good-paying job (finally); no *way* was I going to let my health get in the way.

I ended up learning the hard way that you can never, ever ignore your health. At the time, I was dating the man who would become my husband, and it took him and my mom, and even the patients in the emergency room, to shake some sense into me. For instance, I caught patients staring at my scalp, which was now actively balding. The bold ones asked me point-blank what disease I had or if I had seen a doctor for treatment. Can you imagine? Patients who needed *my* help in an emergency room were telling *me* to get help!

So, I made some appointments. I embarked on the journey—the journey that thousands of my patients have also made. Doctor after doctor listened to me detail my symptoms, and then after an evaluation, they determined I was fine.

There's nothing wrong.

You're stressed.

You're fine.

Over and over, I received the ultimate patronizing dismissal, the biggest lie we women are all told, even though I was a doctor! After the first couple of appointments I thought, *Okay, maybe that was just a bad experience. Let me try again.* Finally, my sixth specialist looked at me, and said, "Young lady, you're probably going to be totally bald in a few years. Here, take this prescription. If you don't, I don't really know what else to do for you."

By that point, I was fed up and furious. Furious at that doctor with a bedside manner of Attila the Hun. Furious at all the other doctors who couldn't be bothered. And furious at myself for not having any solutions. But I didn't know what else to do, because my training was in pediatrics and emergency medicine—plus, I didn't have the time (or so I thought) to do a deep dive into my own health.

I knew I needed to find the root cause of my symptoms, but all those doctors were offering me were Band-Aids. Meanwhile, my hair kept falling out.

So, I took the medicine, which was known to cause a drop in blood pressure. I already had chronically low blood pressure, but none of the six specialists I'd seen had bothered to ask about it. Yes, I'm a doctor. Yes, I should have checked the fine print on the prescription insert for contraindications, but I was already in an emotional funk and I wasn't thinking clearly. After my first dose of the drug in the morning, I went to the gym and worked out, got into my car, and drove off. My blood pressure tanked, I passed out, and I wrecked my car. I came *this* close to hitting other people and putting them (and myself) in danger.

That was it. I was done. *Enough.* In retrospect, I'm grateful to those six patronizing doctors, because their indifference and inability to treat me, coupled with my disappointment in the system in which I was trained, is what completely altered my own attitude and transformed my practice.

I'm going to have to fix this myself, I realized. I started researching for answers. This time I was on my own, fueled by frustration and a determination to heal. After taking time to understand nutrition more deeply, I dove into Ayurvedic and traditional Chinese medicine and soon learned that my debilitating symptoms were likely caused by a *hormonal imbalance that was triggered by emotional stress, trauma, and poor nutrition and lifestyle habits.*

In short, conventional medicine and the one-size-fits-all pharmaceutical approach had failed me; a more holistic approach was needed. I started with resources offered by the American Holistic Health Association, and my mind opened up to a whole new way of thinking. I became even more curious about Eastern systems of medicine, and I pursued certifications in acupuncture and Ayurveda. I studied nutrition, and I completed the requirements to become a certified nutrition specialist. But what really gave me the confidence to practice this different style of medicine was my Integrative Medicine Fellowship with Dr. Andrew Weil. The fellowship opened my mind to the concept of combining different medical thoughts and systems, rather than rely on just one philosophy for all the answers.

For instance, I learned that when you marry traditional Western medicine with other systems of medicine, you gain a powerful formula for not only understanding how to take care of yourself but also how to address all the different aspects of our multiple bodies—emotional, mental, spiritual, physical, and energetic. Merging systems of medicine pulls together the nutrition, lifestyle, and emotional factors, and takes into consideration how they influence human biology—hormones, gut health, and so much more. And as I continued working with patients, I realized that the role of *hormone dysfunction* on overall health was profound: it impacts almost every other system of the body, yet it is routinely missed in practice. And this dismissal, oversight—whatever you want to call it—leaves women feeling confused, defeated, and . . .

old. To every one of those women I gently remind them: *It's not you. It's your hormones!*

How we feel physically directly impacts the communities we hold together—our loved ones and those we influence. What I mean is that if we're walking into our relationships, or our parenting, or the places where we work from this place of feeling *less than*, it has devastating consequences on not only our lives but also the lives of all those we touch. Think about it: How many relationships suffer from the seven-year itch or the eighteen-year slump? Often, those are times of critical hormone shifts occurring in the family. It happens to women with young children usually in their mid-thirties to forties (the perimenopausal years) or to women in their late forties through fifties (in menopause). Is this a coincidence? I don't think so.

Thankfully, women today are fed up with that tired narrative of the "hormonal woman." I see teenagers and pregnant women talking candidly to their friends about their feelings, their first periods, their body changes during pregnancy, and their mood swings. But there is not yet that same openness when women go through perimenopause and menopause. Instead, many women feel like they need to hide, or they keep what they are going through during these phases a secret—something they have guarded and not let out.

I have learned that the road to healing always starts with you—the patient—and where you are along life's journey. By understanding your hormones and the way they change throughout your life, you can also understand the perimenopause and menopause years for what they are: just two of the many shifts that happen. This is never, ever anything to be afraid of or ashamed of; it's just something you need to understand better about your body and your health.

It is a time to be thankful for the lessons, the wins, and the hits—the journey that has brought us all to a place of full arrival. It is a time when women should be celebrated for stepping into their power, for finally receiving their crown, and for assuming their ascension to the throne of queendom. It's your coronation, so to speak.

So, envision yourself coming into your own. Everything else has been a dress rehearsal, or perhaps you have been sitting on the sidelines. But after auditioning once, twice, and maybe even three times, you land the role of leading lady in the drama that is your own life—or at least that is how it should be.

This is your opportunity to claim that power and take the Journey UP. This can only happen, though, if you understand your own hormone story and the influence of those hormones on all aspects of your health. This book is designed to help you do exactly that: to achieve the full expression of your power, to feel incredible in your own skin, to have the best sex of your life, and to radiate your confidence.

Together we will bury the silly stuff that bothered you before. And if you have landed some place where you are not happy, that's okay, too; this book will empower you to push past whatever is holding you back. I've seen so many women truly come into their own, though they had assumed the curtains were down and the show was over. I have watched with the pride of a mentor and the energy of a cheerleader as once-defeated women have found the strength to start companies, write books, create podcasts, end unsatisfying relationships, or make a difference in their communities or underserved areas. And it does not have to be difficult or complicated, as I show you in my Thirty-Day Hormone Reset.

A Holistic Approach to Women's Health

I am here to change the dialogue, the perception, and the conversation about women's health and the hormone shifts all women experience, especially those headed into perimenopause and menopause. This book is not about endings; it's about new beginnings. There's a medical approach in line with this mindset, and it is so much better than what's currently being offered to you.

I *know* there is a better and simpler way. From my own experience and the work done with the 30,000+ patients we have seen in our practices at CentreSpringMD, I've designed a method and a system that works to bring you into hormone balance, that will stabilize your chemistry, and that can help transition you to the next exciting phase of your life.

The methodology I use is a blend of Eastern and Western medicine, and it *works*. It merges the intersecting planes of the body—the emotional, spiritual, physical, hormonal, and mental bodies; it personalizes your body map to raise your vibration and energy levels, providing a solid foundation from which you then make all decisions.

At CentreSpringMD, my job is to hear my patients' stories and then help them draw their own body maps—maps that show how everything fits together. In the process, I stamp out shame and guilt. Then I pull from my expanded medical toolbox multiple systems of medicine to give them the physical results and healing they seek. Most important, I *listen*. And I put a plan in place that acknowledges their issues and provides answers. Finally. This is the way medicine should be.

How do I so easily know that a patient may have adrenal fatigue, or she is low in progesterone, or she is prone to thyroid dysfunction? Eastern systems of medicine stress the importance of effective history taking, energy evaluations, and emotional assessments that point to shifts in a person's biology, which the science and lab work also prove. Many of my patients may start this journey a bit skeptical—*What the heck is she doing?*—but that's okay. As they see the pieces fall into place, with blood tests confirming my diagnosis and supporting the treatment options, that skepticism is often replaced with relief.

What you'll come to learn in this book is that medicine can't be confined to the rigors of the traditional scientific method, because that approach can't take into account every individual's genetics, emotional makeup, generational history, and life experience, as well as how all that shows up in the numbers and chemistry that doctors see in their patients. In short, there are simply too many variables to consider. At the end of the day, if a doctor doesn't take the time to put together all the pieces of a woman's puzzle—by asking not only "What are her lab numbers looking like?" but also "Where is her energy? What's her nutritional bandwidth? What's her hormonal bandwidth?"—then that doctor can't come up with the right solutions.

Consider that traditional Chinese medicine doesn't see the stages of a woman's hormones as having those hard boundaries that Western medicine sees. Chinese medicine sees those hormone levels as fluid, existing on a continuum that a person has a lot of control over—for instance, through diet, quality sleep, personal care, and stress management. A practitioner of Chinese medicine tracks those hormone shifts and works to bring a person back into balance. That's because the shift is not seen as bad; rather, the hormone levels in the body are a marker of a person's *vitality*—they determine if a person is functioning optimally or operating at a deficit.

Does that make you feel better? It should! Hormone management *is* within your control. And mastering your hormones is the secret to feeling your best at any age. And remember—age really is just a number.

What to Expect in This Book

In reading this book you will learn all about hormones in general, the stages of perimenopause and menopause, and the other shifts that happen throughout life. You'll gain practical advice on navigating these stages, and you'll put the pieces of your hormone health together using my Thirty-Day Hormone Reset.

You'll create your own personal body map, which will help you understand how your hormones, diet, and lifestyle influence your emotions, thoughts, and decisions, and vice versa. Together we will rewrite your story and draw a map to follow for your healing and personal discovery. I hope you are as excited about doing this as I am! I cannot wait to hear how your life has been altered as you embrace the guidance offered in these next chapters.

I have divided this book into three major sections, each strategically designed to help you understand the history of hormones and women's health, as well as to change the course of history to herstory—your story.

In Part I, I discuss the history of hormonal treatment, review why women are being gaslit by Western medicine, and explain how to reorient your thinking so you can move forward along the hormone journey—a journey that gets sidelined in kids as young as thirteen. You'll also get a refresher course on the symptoms of hormonal imbalance and learn the ramifications of hormonal shifts over the decades. And you'll learn what the hormones are, as well as the connections between your hormones and your emotions, so as to better understand the why behind your behaviors.

In Part II, I explain the differences between Western and Eastern modalities, and why combining treatments from both kinds of medicine leads to greater success. Know that being open to various medical treatments will give you that wonderfully expanded toolbox for healing. Further, I explain the vital importance of the gut–hormone connection, how hormonal imbalances can affect your emotional state of mind, how to maximize your nutritional choices, and how to clean up your dirty hormones.

In Part III, I set you up to embark on the Thirty-Day Hormone Reset. This is a unique program tailored to correct the most common hormonal imbalances I have seen in my practice. In this program, you'll gain all the information you need to rebalance and reset your hormones for optimal health.

It's been amazingly gratifying to me to see my patients improve. I have watched them glide through the decades of their lives: the roaring twenties, the turbulent thirties, and then perimenopause and menopause. They do it all with none of those dreaded hormone symptoms that have brought women down for generations. These patients are not victims of hot flashes or night sweats, tossing and turning in bed, or sufferers of brain fog, or victims of an overall sense of lost vitality. They live and stand in their power, unapologetically.

Indeed, these women are running marathons, traveling the world, and nurturing themselves and their relationships. *They know how to take care of themselves.* That's what it comes down to. My patients have learned to recognize the factors that influence their hormones and their emotions, and they are treating their bodies with the respect they deserve.

So, commit to healing and understanding your own body, not to "fixing" it—after all, you're not a car. The more nutritional and lifestyle changes you make, the fewer medications you're likely to need across the board, whether they are natural in the form of herbs or other plants or they are pharmaceutical in the form of prescribed pills. If whatever treatment you've been using isn't giving you the results you sought, switch now. Be open to change. Explore different possibilities. And be ready to shift strategies if something isn't working. That's the Journey UP. It's a Journey UP to your greatest powers, your highest self, and your ultimate opportunities. And it's just beginning.

At the risk of sounding hokey, I have seen how getting proper hormonal treatment has opened up the portals of intuition for my patients. I have seen them go from being unable to make a decision or feeling defeated to finding the answers they need for themselves. I hear them say, "Oh, my gosh, like why didn't I think of this before? And now that I know, this is what I'm going to do, and here is what has to change."

Are you ready to rewrite your story? Your body is primed to go. And no, you are never too old to start. The journey to healing doesn't have to be expensive or complicated, or part of a tricky wellness routine. It simply involves marrying the right information with a commitment to YOU.

PART I

Dump the Baggage and Clear the Blockages

chapter 1

The Five Key
Hormone Shifts

Here begins the hormone manifesto that offers information every young girl and woman should understand: how their hormones shift and how to bring them back into balance. So, yes, you can pass this information on to women of all ages: your daughter, mother, sisters, and friends. This is our story, and it's the language we should all be speaking to support, empower, and lead one another across these hormone bridges. This is how we all come together.

Every woman experiences hormonal shifts and disruptions during her lifetime, but the sympathetic nods and offers of help these women got during the roller-coaster years of their puberty seem to disappear with each passing decade, even as the shifts continue to occur. From puberty into early adulthood, to pregnancy and motherhood, and then to perimenopause and menopause, universally there is minimal conversation concerning hormones and hormone shifts, leading women of every age on an endless hunt for answers to "mystery" symptoms and diseases.

What many of these women don't realize is that their hormone journey actually began when they were in their teens and twenties. That's when a foundation of hormone understanding should have been built. Instead, young women are given Band-Aids to manage the shifts (birth control pills, etc.), rather than beginning an exploration into their health. And the result is that more and more young women have hormone-based conditions, including PCOS (polycystic ovarian syndrome), endometriosis, and infertility; fibroids and fibrocystic breast cysts; and many different autoimmune diseases. These conditions are all triggered during a hormone shift. Indeed, this time is the rollercoaster ride that returns for many women decades later, as they enter perimenopause. All of it is there: the anxiety, the crash in self-esteem, even the eating disorders that had been buried—resurfacing as the hormones fluctuate.

The Medical Gaslighting by Mainstream Women's Health

Because these shifts in hormones are poorly understood by mainstream medicine, women have been gaslighted concerning their health, and their hormone symptoms continue to get dismissed in the conversations about their health.

When I graduated from medical school in 1997 and started doing my rotations, the medical field was still a boys' club, to the point of being intimidating. Not only was medicine dominated by male physicians until recently, but the training of medical doctors had limited focus on women's health and hormones. I learned only the basics during my obstetrics/gynecology rotation, and a tiny bit more in the endocrinology rotation (although that delved more into illnesses like diabetes and adrenal disorders). Women and their hormones were viewed in a sort of singular fashion—for either reproduction or their libido—not as a whole-body issue. Have babies and have sex. The END.

So, I'm not angry with any specific doctor, but I am angered by a system that gaslights its patients, spreads the same-old *you're fine* mantra, and keeps women trapped in thinking that we are just getting old or that the problem is all in our heads.

The New Normal

Here is the story the majority of my patients describe: They knew something was *off*, so they went to their primary physician and had lots of blood work done, only to be told their results were "normal." That, really, they were just understandably stressed or anxious or depressed, so they most likely just need an anti-anxiety or anti-depression medication. Or, something for sleep. And something for focus. And something else for weight loss. And yes, there are some side effects, but don't worry about that for now. Because *you're fine.*

That is the "normal" way hormonal symptoms are treated. Women leave their medical visits feeling hopeless, resigned to accepting all their bizarre and unpredictable symptoms. Well, I'm here to tell you that "normal" is not good enough. Historically, "normal" has meant being free of disease; it does not mean *feeling optimal* or *vital* or *vibrant*.

My EastWest holistic approach gets rid of the one-size-fits-all ideology and instead stresses the importance of personal body chemistry and body map. This is the "new normal" that we should all be fighting for. No more bearing the stigma of the "menopausal" or "hormonal" woman, and no more feelings of shame and dread about your hormones and hormone shifts. Women today are demanding and fighting for answers. They are shedding the tired baggage, cleansing it from their psyche, and stepping up to assume their authentic power.

The EastWest approach works *with* our hormones—not against them—to establish balance in all aspects of our bodies—mental, physical, emotional, spiritual, and energetic. But if, instead, you give in to the historic shame and guilt of that gaslighting, know that you are saying no to gifts that await you and power that is rightly yours. This is not your mother's menopause. "Normal" and "fine" do not cut it anymore, and your life story is just beginning, not ending.

What the f*** is happening?

This is a question I hear every day. Women today, at every age, are busy. They are juggling jobs, multitasking, getting lots of things done. And then something changes. They go from super-sharp to foggy, from energetic to tired, or from happy to sad. The hormone shifts that women experience can catch them by surprise, and they can leave them feeling, well, not like themselves anymore.

The hormone journey is one of hormone shifts—except we just don't talk about it. But knowledge is power. Knowing what's happening takes away the fear of the unknown; it arms a woman with the tools to move forward. Understanding the hormone shifts that happen at certain points in a woman's life—whether young girl, teen, young adult, mother, or grandmother—prepares her for what she will need to feel her best. We don't drive cars without some instruction or start careers without some training or education, right? Then why would our bodies be any different? Part of that preparation is not just recognizing the hormone shifts but also understanding what those hormones are and how they play together.

If you are reading this book, you may think you are too young or too old to have a hormone imbalance. You may have been conditioned into believing that life is being in a state of what I call Hormone Hell, that PMS (premenstrual syndrome), abdominal pain, hot flashes, brain fog, or disrupted sleep—to name just a few symptoms—is completely normal.

The journey our hormones make mirrors the phases of our lives as women. Think back to your teen years. Do you remember the highs and lows, the extreme emotions, the new physical symptoms you had to get used to? You most likely nod your head, remembering with empathy that teen version of yourself, when you were flooded with hormones that made you boy crazy, moody, and volatile with your parents (and even your friends). This was your first hormone shift. And if it threw you off balance then, why are you surprised when you are thrown off balance in perimenopause? That's your third hormone shift.

Do you ignore the shift? You can try, but your body will not let you. Instead of nudging you into the role of your lifetime, you are stuck in a walk-on part or even on the sidelines. And you feel trapped. That's because you don't feel good. You don't feel like yourself. And that is not what's meant for you to be.

Yet hormone shifts are a natural part of every woman's story—it's a story that we should know by heart. Indeed, these shifts are nothing new or novel, though women today remain in the dark about them, as are their doctors. You may have been in perimenopause years before any symptoms showed up, or you may have resigned yourself to the unpleasant mood swings, hot flashes, or other symptoms—without ever realizing you don't have to suffer from them.

I am passionate that women understand their hormones. It's a conversation that applies to all women and girls, from the age of thirteen on up. So, I identify here the five key hormone shifts that all women should all be aware of.

1. The Rock Star Shift: Why Thirteen Is as Important as Thirty

Ages 13–19
Key word: Confusion

I love young women of this age so much, but misinformation has convinced them they know it all. (After all, it's on TikTok, right?) Dazed and confused, many girls I see assume it's totally normal to skip periods, and it's even better to not have a period at all. They think that birth control pills are the only way to regulate their hormones. Or, they believe that painful cramps, mood swings, and bloating are an inevitable (and debilitating) part of the game—that there's nothing they can do about it. "You're turning into a woman, right? Welcome! Welcome to Hormone Hell."

There's no reason for a young woman of this age to suffer through the "growing pains" of adolescence just because she's a girl. Most teens don't think their hormones need to be checked, and most moms of teens don't even think blood work is necessary—*and neither do most pediatricians.*

The foundation for our hormones is laid in the teen years. Often, this is when a girl's hormone journey begins, so if issues are dismissed in the exam room when they are actually essential to the girl's overall hormonal balance, it's like putting a bandage on a bullet hole. We have to prepare them for their hormonal shifts, and we have to see them through those shifts—and trust me, that isn't easy!

My own daughter went through this. When she turned thirteen, she started having some issues, and I didn't know how much was the typical teen stuff of finding herself and how much was her hormones. Like all young teens, she was self-conscious, but she wanted to copy her peers when it came to solving issues I knew had a hormonal root. For example, she wanted Accutane for acne, Ritalin for ADHD (attention deficit hyperactivity disorder), and something else to stop her period. If only her friends were talking about the root cause of these issues—that it was hormones and an overall hormone imbalance. No luck there, as you can imagine. I had to learn to smile and nod (so hard, FYI).

It took some convincing, but I did manage to get my daughter's hormone levels checked. Her blood work showed higher than normal levels of androgens, which had led to polycystic ovarian syndrome (PCOS) and possible early endometriosis. This massive fluctuation in her hormone levels inflamed her moods and affected her ability to focus. I started treating her with gentle diet modification and herbs to clean her liver and lower the amount of yeast that lives in the digestive system. (I promise more on that later.) She had the classic "dirty liver," causing "dirty hormones," which led to her symptoms. (More on that later, too.)

Both her experience and mine much earlier are not unlike those of so many teens who never get diagnosed properly, and who suffer hormone issues or conditions like PCOS until finally diagnosed much later. They live (and suffer) the symptoms and issues for decades, not feeling well. I have treated women in perimenopause and menopause who tell me their stories, and I know they had PCOS in their teen years. So much heartache and confusion and expense could have been spared if the condition had been diagnosed early, in this first hormone stage.

The Basics of Puberty

Puberty is the hormonally triggered dividing line between a child's body and a woman's body. Triggered by the pituitary gland, estrogen levels start to increase so that sexual development can begin. Every girl's body is different, and there's no way to predict when puberty might start or how long it might take.

Medically, the changes are defined by what's called the *Tanner stages*. Stage 1 shows no development; stages 2 to 4 track the changes in breast development, hair growth on the body, bone growth, curvature of the hips, and skin changes (such as acne or oiliness). By stage 4, usually around the age of twelve or thirteen, a girl will get her first period. And by stage 5, the breasts reach their approximate adult size and shape, growth stops, the hip area fills out, her periods should be regular, and the reproductive organs and genitals are fully developed.

Precocious Puberty

Many parents of young girls are worried about *precocious puberty*, which describes hormonal changes that arrive earlier than average—even in a girl as young as eight or nine. Those parents are right to be worried, as there's an emotional risk; obviously, there's also a psychosocial risk (the big difference in maturity between a nine-year-old and a thirteen-year-old), and there's just a pure health risk. That is, girls who go into early puberty tend to have more problems with weight gain, inflammation, and growth suppression. Early puberty can also affect the growth rate, as girls tend to stop growing about two years after they get their first period. Plus, the fact that a ten-year-old who's getting her period has to deal with that situation during the school day and can suffer physical symptoms, as well as embarrassment if she gets teased.

I'm often asked if there's a connection between precocious puberty and an earlier ending to the fertile years. I don't think there's a direct link, which is a relief, as every woman's hormonal makeup is different. But I do believe that precocious puberty can be triggered by environmental issues—that is, the sum of what a child eats and the nutrient levels, lifestyle, electronic exposure, sleep quality, and environmental toxins, such as those found in plastics, parabens, phthalates, organophosphates, and more, as well as body care, air, and water. All these can lead to estrogen levels that are much higher than normal—a.k.a. dirty estrogen.

Precocious puberty *can* be slowed down. Mainstream medicine's approach might be to go right to hormone blockers, but they can have side effects. (Rapid onset of precocious puberty should be supervised by a pediatric endocrinologist.) I prefer less drastic measures and concentrate on cleaning up the liver to calm it down and rid the body of toxins—which has worked in my practice.

Dirty Hormones Start Here

We expect teens to be moody—they are trying to figure out their place in the world, right? But there is, trust me, a difference between moodiness and full-out anxiety, depression, OCD (obsessive compulsive disorder), or self-harm; and yes, many of these conditions are hormonally influenced.

This means testing the girl's hormones at least yearly and identifying the troubling hormone patterns I am seeing in my practice. Here is what I am most concerned about:

- Elevated androgens (the sex hormones): high levels of DHT (dihydrotestertone), testosterone, DHEA (dehydroepiandrosterone), free testosterone
- Insulin sensitivity
- Estrogen dominance (storage of estradiol and estrone)

It's not just girls—boys should have their hormones tested as well. Owing to inflammation (which you'll read about in more detail in Part II), there can be an estrogenization of boys' hormones, just as there can be an androgenization of girls' hormones. That leaves boys walking around with more belly fat, mood instability, and insulin resistance, while girls have high testosterone that shows up as acne, hair loss, excess body hair, and mood swings.

There are a lot of theories about the root causes of teenage hormonal imbalances. Hormonal fluctuations are par for the course in adolescence, but the extremes we are experiencing in this generation are troubling. The hormone crisis actually begins at this stage and then perpetuates and exaggerates in the ensuing decades.

Why is this happening? Food quality is going down, while body fat is going up. Our toxic environment is weighing down the gut and the liver. Stress affects our children as well; they are overscheduled, overfed with poor-quality food, not sleeping enough, not getting enough sunlight, and never seem to play outside in nature anymore.

Why Hormones Matter in Our Teenagers

One word: *inflammation.* Not in a joint or a muscle but as an all-over angry fire that engulfs your adorable daughter or son and turns them into aliens from another planet—if fact, you would not mind sending them back to that planet. (No personal experience here . . . !)

Hormones drive inflammation. It's a fundamental concept in the world of integrative and functional medicine, and it's one we need our teens to understand right now. Many children are entering their hormonal years already inflamed—yet they should *not* be suffering from inflammatory conditions that can be prevented by diet and lifestyle changes. They already have higher blood sugar levels, higher insulin levels, more body weight, and more gut dysfunction than children of previous generations. But add the hormones. Add the usual adolescent challenges (Who are my friends? Who am I? Why are these my parents?). And say hello to mental health issues like anxiety and depression, learning challenges, and poor risk-taking and decision-making skills.

This is one of the reasons the obesity epidemic in this country is so scary. So many young girls have estrogen levels that are too high or progesterone levels that are too low for their age. When a child enters that hormone journey already inflamed—which is what obesity essentially does to the body—and the hormone shifts start, anxiety and depression can take over, leading to eating disorders, academic failures, and worse.

Here's the bottom line: teenagers should have their hormone levels checked at least once a year. Go more often if there are any problems such as super-heavy periods, irregular periods, or symptoms of PCOS. This annual record will establish a baseline so that future levels can be checked against previous years, and that will divulge any patterns that might need to be addressed as these teens get older. And please do this before your teenager starts on birth control.

Let's Talk About Your Child's Period

In Eastern medicine, the period is seen as a sign of vitality or health, not as a nuisance or a burden; getting that regular period is really important.

In Western medicine, however, it's all about the dodge. How do you get rid of it? How do you hide it? I've heard girls tell me they're glad they're not getting their period regularly, because bleeding is so gross.

That's an incredibly unhealthy attitude. A regular monthly period means your teen's female hormones are balanced and functioning as they should be. But our society sets extreme thinness as the gold standard of feminine beauty and acceptability, and girls who are extremely thin are unlikely to have normal hormone levels. I've had "The Talk" too many times with teens and their parents about the dangers of sacrificing one's health to lose weight. We joke about calling the period "Auntie Flow," but then I point out that "Auntie" also sounds like *Anti*—as in being anti your normal bodily functions as a female. Instead, I want every girl and woman to embrace the fact that getting your period is not something to dread.

That Least Favorite Monthly Topic: PMS

The headaches. The bloating. The mood swings. Oh, those wretched, painful cramps! No wonder women call their period *the curse.*

Part of why women dread getting their periods is that it just plain hurts. But there's no reason any teen should believe she is doomed to a lifetime of monthly agony. There is a way forward to rid yourself of painful PMS. For instance, it can be improved by simply cleaning up your teen's diet and balancing her nutrients. You'll learn more about this in Chapter 9 when we go over the Thirty-Day Hormone Reset.

The point is that understanding the hormone chemistry, rather than trying to block or superficially treat it, is the best strategy—at any age. The sooner we all do this, the better—whether we are thirteen or sixty-five.

The Pros and Cons of Birth Control

The default method for teens planning to be sexually active used to be the birth control pill, but the conventional default of late is to get an IUD (intrauterine device). This is a better option, as an IUD still secretes some hormones (some versions have progesterone), but those levels are far below the kind of hormonal disruption caused by the pill. It is very difficult to get pregnant when using either the pill or an IUD, although antibiotics can influence the pill's effect if both pills need to be taken at the same time.

The pill is designed to alter the hormone levels so pregnancy doesn't result. It dramatically suppresses the body's production of estrogen, progesterone, and testosterone so there's no ovulation. Unfortunately, there's no way to predict how the pill might make someone feel. Some women do fine on it, especially if they've had super-heavy periods and intense PMS symptoms for years. They lose weight and have more energy. Other women can get depressed, anxious, or feel nauseous all the time. They can gain weight. And the liver burden—yes, an Eastern concept—is a setup for future health issues.

These latter symptoms tend to be worse with birth control shots and implants, since the body is loaded with heavier doses of hormones. Plus, you're not looking at hormone metabolites to see whether your body is processing them effectively or not. Detoxing—the body's ability to remove dirty hormones or toxic metabolites of hormones—is a universal concept, applicable to all ages of women (and men—but that's a different book!).

My EastWest approach to hormone balancing allows for more options. If a teenager—or a woman of any age—is having incredibly painful periods that she can't get under control through diet, lifestyle, or herbal or supplement interventions, then birth control absolutely is an option. As long as you understand that it's a temporary fix because it does not address the root cause of some of these symptoms.

My recommendation for a young woman who is considering birth control is to try an IUD first. Understand, though, that the IUD doesn't protect against STDs (sexually transmitted diseases), that it may cause weight gain and water retention, and that some users experience additional symptoms. The copper in some IUDs and the progesterone in others can also be problematic for certain patients.

If the IUD isn't an option, I suggest going to the lowest hormonally dosed pill as the next option. For the short term, it should be okay. Problems arise when women have been on the pill for more than five years and are using the pill for hormone balance rather than for birth control. I always say that birth control pills should be used only for birth control—not for hormone balancing.

Set Your Teen for Hormonal (and All Other) Success

If your teenage daughter has terrible hormonal symptoms, is that a sign she's likely to have them again later in life, especially if they aren't addressed now? Yes, unfortunately! So, if you do have a teenage girl, NOW is the time to start her hormone journey. That's because it's our job as mothers to try to get our girls set up for success, not just for today but also for their twenties and beyond.

The Rock Star's Top Three Checklist
1. Get blood work done every twelve months to check on hormone levels. (For specifics, see page 124 in Chapter 3.)

2. Embrace the period as a vital sign. A power sign.

3. Determine the best diet, exercise routine, and overall wellness plan that keeps your cycle happy and healthy, rather than causing you to retreat and withdraw. But if you are withdrawing, getting anxious, feel depressed, or are moody, go back to #1 here, or see your medical provider to dig deeper into these issues.

2. The Hustler Shift: Dating, Career Building, and Finding Yourself

Ages 20-28
Key word: Invincible

Invincible. That's how you feel. You've now got that independence, and it's time to make your mark in the world. You're working it, busting it, and trying to make it big in all areas of your life—school, work, finances, relationships (oh, the relationships!).

This is also the decade when you're not just busting it but also burning the candle at both ends. You're staying out late and partying hard. You think you're never going to be any way other than how you are at this moment. You have a sense that you're invincible, right? Because you have time on your side.

But if you're hustling too hard, you may start to miss periods, experience sudden weight loss or gain, develop acne, suffer hair loss, or feel anxiety—you name it. Your first instinct might be to slap a temporary bandage on these symptoms and push through. But pause for a moment: *your body is trying to tell you something.*

Keeping Up with Other Hustlers

It's all in the hustle; and yes, now is the time to prove yourself. I should know, as I used to be like you—staying up late, waking up early, partying when time allowed, being totally financially strapped and stressed, and constantly navigating family dramas and medical school stress. Why was I surprised that my hair fell out, my joints were swollen, and I gained weight? My lifestyle and choices were ripe for Hormone Hell.

Fast-forward twenty years, and the pressure on young women continues to increase. Social media has left us all more looks-obsessed and self-conscious, while the increase in mental health disorders means that the majority of Hustlers are on some prescription medicine; further, some go on to abuse those medications. Then, sprinkle in a new age of relationships and dating patterns, along with a growth in virtual work, and the Hustlers now not only are stressed but also are isolated.

This is the decade when it all starts to fall apart. When young women are told that everything is fine, that the birth control pill or IUD will solve their hormone issues, and any mood or mental health issues just need—well, you guessed it—another medication.

But it should not be this way. This time of your life is very much still a foundational decade, a time to focus on health and wellness, because anyone past the age of twenty-eight knows that life just gets even busier. So, what do I want you all to do? Get those hormones checked again, keep those medical appointments with doctors who have a holistic approach, and know your numbers. Think about optimizing for the future rather than just about living in the here and now.

In my practice, I most often see the following hormone patterns and/or conventional diagnosis in Hustlers:

- PCOS (polycystic ovarian syndrome)
- Endometriosis (when the uterine lining grows outside of the uterus, often undiagnosed)
- POTS (postural orthostatic tachycardia syndrome, a blood circulation disorder)
- Anovulatory cycle (no ovulation)
- Dysmenorrhea (intense pain and cramps during your period)
- PMDD (premenstrual dysphoric disorder, involving severe and long-lasting PMS)
- Hashimoto's thyroiditis (an autoimmune disease of the thyroid gland)

The hormone patterns that accompany these diagnoses include:

- Low progesterone levels
- High androgens: DHT/androstenedione/testosterone, total and free
- High insulin, Hgb A1C, C-peptide, insulin levels
- High levels of the stress hormone cortisol, which can cause weight gain, trouble sleeping, anxiety, and depression
- Thyroid issues, which usually become noticeable after the age of twenty-five and include a wide range of symptoms that disrupt metabolism and cognitive functioning
- Internal inflammation, leading to slow but inexorable development of autoimmune conditions

You'll learn more about all these hormones matters in Chapter 3.

Be a Wise Hustler.

Listen up, Hustlers. I was once one of you, and this is when I started to get into real trouble because I didn't have a clue what was going on. I had no idea that young women who emerge from adolescence feeling stressed or with trauma will find their hormones going haywire as they enter their twenties.

Why does this happen? Eastern systems of medicine, including Chinese and Ayurvedic medicine, teach us that stress and anger are stored in the liver, while fear and worry are held in the kidneys and spleen. All these organ and meridian systems regulate hormones and influence disease (more about meridians in Chapter 4). For instance, the liver is critical for hormone breakdown and detoxification, while the gut determines how hormones are metabolized and packaged. This is why stress triggers heavy periods, or why too many sleepless nights contribute to insulin resistance (and, therefore, belly fat), or why too many nights being hungover lead to high testosterone and androgen levels (with subsequent acne or hair loss).

These connections are why I am passionate about members of this age group; I wish someone had given me this information back then, or shook me and shouted, "Hey, Ms. Hustler—I want you to pay attention to this stuff!"

If you don't want to get pregnant, you may very well be thinking about your hormones strictly in terms of birth control. If you're sexually active, you can't just think about dating or STDs (sexually transmitted diseases), or having a loving partner. You also need to think about the actual physical functioning and chemistry of your body. Again, your body and your hormones are talking to you—*please listen!*

Of course, a lot of Hustlers take their health for granted. They're young, they're vibrant, they have no issues even when taking minimal care of themselves. Of course, if you're feeling good and have a menstrual cycle that works like clockwork, it is not unreasonable to think that nothing is wrong. But in reality there may be something wrong—you may not be "fine."

It's very easy to not listen to your body because you're busy hustling, and it's easier to assume nothing is wrong. You power through the days and nights, while attributing any changes to just being super-busy or super-tired. Instead, think of this time as a chance to pay attention to anything that looks bad (like your skin) or that feels bad (like your PMS or your joints). Understand how you feel, analyze what you are eating and drinking, and even consider what you are eliminating.

I have this conversation all the time with women in their twenties. That's because they've got so much going on in their lives that they tend to downplay their symptoms until they develop a full-on health crisis. As I once did. But this is the decade when you've got to throw the *of course* out the window and become a mother to your own self. As in, take care of your wonderful body right now, and prepare for the future. By really digging into your health, you are on the Journey UP.

What does that mean? You need to know your genetics, your nutrients, and your hormone levels. You can then stabilize your gut health and lower your risk of inflammation. You will understand your toxic load and what that means for your long-term health—and even for your future children. You put the pieces of your puzzle together.

This really does matter for your life, both now and in the future, and so this is what we are going to do in the next few chapters. Part of this journey involves tracking your hormone patterns and levels. That is, I want you ahead of, and not behind, the hormone game. I want you fully aware of when things can go haywire, so you can catch yourself before some ill-informed doctor tells you that you have low ovarian reserve, or you must try to get pregnant right away, or you need a shelf full of expensive medications to manage those mystery symptoms.

Ignoring your hormones and your health now will unfortunately set you up for bigger problems in the future. No matter how stressed you are at work, or how busy you are in your life, or how much fun you're having, put your hormones—and your health—on your to-do list. Keeping track of your hormone levels now also means you'll be in excellent shape should you decide to become pregnant soon or later in your thirties, when your fertility naturally begins to decline. Be the best Hustler you can by building the strongest possible foundation for your future hormonal health.

The Hustler's Top Three Checklist

1. Have a full hormone panel and inflammation test done every twelve months. (For specifics about which tests to get, see page 124.) See your gynecologist once a year for a Pap smear, breast exam, and to address any gynecological concerns; also see your primary care doctor for an evaluation of hormones and inflammation markers. (Most if not all these lab tests should be covered by your medical insurance, which, yes, you need to have.)

2. Burning the candles at both ends will soon burn you up and send your hormones into Overwhelm status. Do an inventory of all the things that may be causing you stress—and be honest! Start investigating and incorporating stress-busting techniques into your day.

3. Realize that if you ignore hormone problems now, they won't go away.

3. The Superstar Shift: Answering the Call of Nature

Ages 29–38

Key word: Frazzled!

Full-out juggler mode begins right here. Are you ready? Or rather, are your hormones ready to morph from a Hustler to a Superstar?

During this phase, your big life goals get real—really fast. That's particularly true for those women who want to enter committed relationships or who are looking for one, and certainly if they are hoping to have children. The Superstar years are when the pull of managing a household, a family, or a busy career might start to tip the health and hormonal balance, and you end up frazzled.

The majority of my patients are having their first babies when they are in their thirties or their second child when they are into their forties. This is a noticeable shift from the pattern one or two generations ago, when the average life span was shorter, women got married younger (in part because they had fewer career options), and cultural standards were to start a family right after marriage. While there are so many more options for women now, the biological fact is inescapable: your fertility starts to decline when you are in your thirties. So, at this point in your life you may be trying to get pregnant, to stay pregnant, to breastfeed, to get pregnant again, or to freeze your eggs for future use. I'm exhausted just thinking about all this, as I remember how shattered I was when this phase happened to me. It occurred all while I was trying to maintain my career and find a few minutes in the day for self-care. No wonder our word for Superstars is *frazzled*.

I have found that so many women who enter this phase unprepared, as I did, assume that motherhood and maintaining a work-life balance would be easy, seamless. After all, hadn't we just been the Hustlers, who busted it through our twenties unscathed? We are still full of energy and plans and goals, and we can multitask like fiends.

Many of my Superstar patients also tell me they are surprised at how lonely they feel in their thirties. Even if they are in a loving partnership, this is the age when there's a shift in your social groups. That is, your childhood friends have scattered. Your high school buddies have moved on. Your college buddies are now doing their own thing. Your mommy friends are crazy-busy with their families. If most of your friends are married and you're not, you can feel very alone, like the stereotypical third wheel. Or, you've had to move somewhere new for work and you haven't made a lot of new friends, so there's the subsequent loneliness.

The truth, unfortunately, is that it's not easy or simple to wear the many hats we women are expected to wear today. Ultimately, our hormones rebel, tired of ongoing demands to push through and move forward, without replenishment. Sooner or later, there is a price to pay in the hormone world, whether it's estrogen dominance, thyroid instability, unexplained weight gain, or any series of other unwanted symptoms.

Common Hormone Patterns for Superstars

I've found that stress is the main culprit for many of the hormonal issue facing Superstars.

I got married when I was thirty-two, had my daughter when I was thirty-four, opened my practice when I was thirty-five, and had my son when I was thirty-six. It was an incredible birthing phase for me, personally and professionally. I look back on those days fondly, but with a big caveat. My daughter was looking at photos of all of us from those days, and the first thing she said was, "You look *so* tired!" Oh, was I tired. Or rather, utterly exhausted. I was taking care of two kids under fifteen months of age with a new practice and a hospital job. I was *frazzled*.

I did what many women do during this phase of life: I worked really long days, moving from task to task without taking a breath. I went to bed at 3 a.m. (my team remembers those 2 a.m. emails). I also wanted to enjoy every minute of my kids when they were little and totally adorable, but it was often hard because I was so stressed and exhausted. I wanted to complete the next task, thinking the list would somehow get shorter as a result. I was so frazzled that I've lost years from that time—honestly, I don't remember them at all. Talk about the bitter with the sweet!

In other words, this is the phase when Superwoman syndrome appears. Too often, though, we ignore the signs because we don't yet have the maturity to let some things go and to calm down. A Superwoman feels she has to be super all the time—there's no Off switch. She tries to reach her goals both emotionally and energetically, and if she doesn't reach them, there can be a little bit of panic.

Realize, as well, that if you had a pretty tumultuous time as a Hustler, your thirties will not be a vacation, and health issues and hormone disruption are common. A lot of my patients think this disorder is due to their genetic makeup, but genes play only a minor role compared to the stressors and strains of your daily life. For example, my patient Susannah had a mother who, it turned out, had an MTHFR deficiency (methylenetetrahydrofolate reductase), a mutation that can cause various clotting disorders, cardiovascular diseases, and a drive toward inflammation, causing her mom to have a history of frequent miscarriages. Not knowing why she'd lost so many pregnancies, she told Susannah to hurry up and have babies early, just in case. But Susannah was not ready to get pregnant, so I suggested she get genetic testing to rule out any potential problems. When the results arrived, Susannah was relieved to see she was perfectly normal, while her mother was shocked to learn that she had MTHFR. They had made incorrect assumptions because they didn't have all the information they needed.

Superstars will find that their hormones at this time are about to shift. Thirty-five is the average age when the first perimenopausal symptoms begin, when estrogen and progesterone levels start their slow decline (which is absolutely normal). At first, that shift is subtle. It's not a steep downhill decline; rather, there's a gradual diminishment until you feel it impacting your life. Impacting how you feel and impacting how you see yourself. Maybe you'll have your first episode of brain fog; you'll find yourself standing in your dining room, wondering why you came in and what you are looking for. Maybe you won't rebound as quickly as before after a hard workout. Maybe you'll notice a little bit of belly fat that wasn't there before. Or, you'll experience mid-cycle spotting, and your periods will fluctuate from light one month to more frequent for a few months, then back to light again.

Then, when your progesterone levels start to go down even a little bit, you might become more anxious. You can lose sleep; that's because progesterone acts as a checks-and-balances system for cortisol. So, if you've had a high cortisol level for years, your normal levels of progesterone were helping you manage those cortisol levels, allowing you to sleep through stress or whatever else you were dealing with. All of a sudden, now you're up at 4 a.m. and then the alarm goes off at 6 a.m. Your tossing and turning has left you virtually sleepwalking, in a fog.

Or, you're up and staring at the ceiling between 2 and 4 a.m., so you don't wake up in the morning feeling refreshed. Most of my patients tell me that when this happens, they just keep on powering through—until the exhaustion finally catches up with them.

In addition, when your estrogen levels start to fluctuate, the hot flashes, achy joints, brain fog, mood swings, and more can appear. Your periods may become extremely heavy and irregular. Many women start to gain weight, particularly in their hips, thighs, or abdomen. In response, they often work out harder, but since that doesn't work, they do even more intense cardio sessions.

If you have any of these symptoms, denial is not your friend. At this stage, women can be pretty bad at figuring out what's going on or keeping track of their symptoms and fluctuations. Instead of being frazzled, you need to establish a relationship with a physician who is willing to dig deep into your health status and understands how to not only treat an illness but also keep you well and vital. After all, you can truly care for all those around you and accomplish your goals. We will be doing this together in the course of this book.

The Time to Get Pregnant Is Now

One of the most heartbreaking conversations I have—and it's one I have too often—is with women who are unable to become pregnant just when they most desperately want to. Perhaps because of circumstances, they weren't able to try for a baby when they were younger, or perhaps they met the love of their life later and were now ready to have that baby—but it is too late for their eggs. You can still be fertile during perimenopause, but untreated hormone imbalances make conception and carrying a baby to term much harder, especially when it is discovered late in the game. That's also why all women who become pregnant at the age of thirty-five or later are defined as having "advanced maternal age." Now, doesn't that term make you feel old? It shouldn't, but that doesn't mean you can pretend your body isn't changing.

If you were tracking your hormones year to year, any nuances in hormone balance would have been caught earlier, making natural fertility more realistic. This is why I've included that information in the book (see page 124); this is the decade when Superstars need to assess their current life situation, along with their hopes and dreams for the future. Does that dream include children? What is the path forward? Knowing your hormones as you enter this decade is the first step toward determining that future.

Reproductive technology has given millions of women the ability to have children when they couldn't get pregnant naturally, but this option takes a serious toll on your body at any age. I have a patient who at fifty-five is trying to get pregnant. She had harvested her eggs when she was much younger, and she had one successful pregnancy. Now, along with her reproductive endocrinologist, I am helping her manage her hormones. But her body is in revolt; her thyroid gland is now out of control, as she's had to take megadoses of hormones to maintain the pregnancy, and she suffers jaundice because her liver and gall bladder are stressed. What is the fallout from all of this? We are still learning.

An experienced reproductive endocrinologist can give you more advice about what procedures might work for you, and there is no shame in exploring all your options. But the bottom line is this: Know your hormones. Know your body. Know how fertile you are so as to avoid unnecessary stress.

Managing the Superstar Stress

Want to know what is one of the biggest fertility blocks? Stress. The List. The simple goal of "I am going to get pregnant." It's a goal approached with a singular focus, which the body then rejects. Sit down and take a deep breath. The smartest thing you can do is to get your hormone levels tested at least once a year. Regularly reassess your energy level. Also, establish routines. For instance, you need a good night's sleep. You need to know that you do *not* have to do everything that is asked of you.

As a Superstar, I learned through suffering and a whole lot of stress that the most important word you will utter during this decade is *no*. Women are really bad at saying that word. Instead, find your voice and speak up. Ask for help when you need it, delegate to others, and tell yourself you can't do it all.

This is the warning bell, ringing loud, for women who enter or want to be entering motherhood, and are doing so at the time when their careers are starting to pick up and become more demanding, with more responsibilities and less free time. Remember, you can't do it all. Or, rather, you can try to do it all, but eventually something will snap and you'll crash. Finding that sweet spot, that point of balance, to minimize the stress that then shows up in your hormone levels can be really, really tough. For women who are single, the stress of not being in a relationship might hit particularly hard, most especially if they want to have children. The biological clock is ticking loudly enough to rival Big Ben.

What you need now is a plan. This is absolutely not the time to say, "I'll deal with this later," because later never comes. I've been guilty of this myself. I don't have time for my health right now. I've got babies.

I've got a business. I've got all this other stuff going on, you know? Just remember that "later" needs to be *today*, because tomorrow can be costly.

While this third hormonal shift is a shake-up time, don't see it in a negative light. See it as the time when you can shake it up for good, clarify your goals, and have the inner strength not only to go for it but also to find your own voice. You should now be savvy enough and honest enough with yourself to do that self-check, quickly and efficiently. Know when you're getting into trouble, identify the causes, and have that roadmap for taking care of your hormones.

The Superstar's Top Three Checklist
1. Practice saying no until it's as easy as saying hello.
2. Faithfully get your hormone levels checked annually (see page 124), and if you are having trouble getting pregnant, or want to get pregnant in the future, obtain expert advice about your options.
3. Add as many stress-busting techniques as you can to your daily routine. (For more on this, see Chapter 4.)

4. The Superwoman Shift: Owning Your Power

Ages 39–55
Key Word: Authenticity

When you turned forty-six, did you look in the mirror and say to yourself, *Hey, where did all those wrinkles come from? How can this be? In my head I'm still a twentysomething Hustler!*

With all those amazing Superwomen out there, doing amazing things, these years should be a celebration of all they have accomplished, refined, learned, and created. As one of them, you've earned the right to no longer be thought of as a twinkling Superstar but, now, as a true Superwoman. I know you can look and feel every bit the part, even if you might start to feel that those great days are behind you.

Here's the deal: This fourth phase is a critical one for women—a time when illnesses or diseases can often first show up, and the sum of our adventures from previous decades hands us a health report card that may or may not be to our liking. (I wrote about the very real Superwoman syndrome in my 2017 book *The Superwoman Rx*.) This is also a time of dramatically shifting hormone levels, when the arrival of perimenopause and then menopause looks or feels like a midlife crisis. Maybe you're used to being full of energy and not needing much sleep . . . and then suddenly a stressor (your family or your work situation changes) arrives and you can't manage things like you once did. You don't have the same energy level, but you think you do, so you will yourself into believing and try to power through. The symptoms start hitting you and it feels like they're controlling you, rather than the other way around. One of my patients summarized it perfectly: "I'm itchy and bitchy!"

We can't be blasé about this, thinking, *Well, you know, yeah, it's no big deal that my periods are getting kind of irregular or I feel more tired all the time. Maybe I'm just* off, *you know, because I've got so much going on. No biggie, right?* Wrong! I've yet to meet a woman who, without advice and treatment from a medical professional, had absolutely no perimenopausal symptoms, breezing through these years without a speck of worry. It's gonna happen, and my job is to get you ready for it, so you do feel that calming breeze instead of being hit with a major hurricane.

Now more than ever, Superwomen need to confront and change the trajectory of conversations that might be happening with their regular doctors. If your symptoms are being diminished or dismissed, no, they are not in your head. And no, you are not just "getting old."

You don't have to listen to the insulting "Sorry, but you should suck it up and endure them" or "You're fine" spiels. Instead, it's mandatory you take a proactive approach to your overall health and your hormone health.

So much of what you may feel and experience during these years is reversible—if and when you establish and follow your own personalized roadmap to wellness. Superwomen should have confidence that they're going to be living longer than women of previous generations. Doing so gives you the time to make the changes you need to make, whether you do it in incremental shifts or an enormous leap into a totally new lifestyle.

Common Hormone Issues for Superwomen

As discussed in the preceding Superstar section, perimenopause is the time when those annoying symptoms—hot flashes, night sweats, irregular cycles, fatigue, anxiety, depression, intense moodiness, disrupted sleep, and weight gain—arrive, and it's usually when you least expect or want them. The dysregulation of cortisol, our stress hormone, can go haywire even before your estrogen and progesterone levels start to drop. You might notice that your tolerance of stress changes. Perhaps you were proud of how well you could juggle dozens of projects at a time, but now the slightest hitch is taking you near the edge. Those Hustler days when you went away for a fun weekend and arrived back home as the sun was about to rise, then you showered and got to work knowing that a few large lattes would see you through the day—well, those times are a distant memory (maybe, you have to admit, that is not always a *bad* thing.).

Or maybe you just don't feel that great and you don't know why, and that feeling starts to bleed into your relationships and into your work. Your family and friends might be dropping hints. If so, that likely causes a little bit of a spiral. You feel so crummy that you start self-soothing to make the discomfort go away. You find yourself eating the wrong stuff, so you gain weight. You're frustrated that you're gaining weight, and that makes you feel less sexy. Your libido disappears. You start to feel foggy.

An incremental slowing down of your body's systems is a normal part of aging, and it explains why Superwomen can find it that much harder to do things that used to be easy—those things that have always kept you fit and healthy. Know that this slowing down is connected to the slight decline in your hormone levels. The rate of muscle building lowers; digestion gets a bit more sluggish; and your immune system has to work harder to protect you. If your progesterone level is dropping, you're going to crave more salt. If your estrogen level is low, you're hunting for fats to fuel you. If your thyroid levels are off, you'll have other cravings. If your iron's low, you'll often want sugar to buy energy. This hormonal decline often drives behaviors that result in unwanted weight gain, anxiety, and depression.

Your forties are either a call for truth serum or a mirror reflecting how you have lived the last twenty years. You might have lived hard, partied hard, got stressed, had trauma, got divorced, lost this, mourned that. If so, you can have it rough as you feel the toll these times have taken. If they remain unchecked, your hormone imbalances can turn extreme, the autoimmune disorders suddenly appear and the belly fat won't go away. Not that the toll isn't reversible, but it declares itself unremittingly. You can't hide from the truth anymore. And if you don't acknowledge it, your body will *force* you to acknowledge it. This is the time to reframe the next twenty years of your life.

Men Have Hormonal Issues, Too

Believe me when I say that a lot of relationships fall apart owing to shifting hormone levels, not only in women but also in men!

It's fair to generalize that men tend to be less in tune with their hormones because they don't have monthly hormonally driven cycles or drastic hormonal shifts on a regular basis in their lives. They can empathize with women having painful PMS, but they don't live with the symptoms. Men only realize that they might have hormonal issues if they're having trouble in the bedroom, especially a loss of libido. Or they experience cognitive changes, especially if they're dealing with a lot of stress. A lot of them also suffer in silence, or get irritable and snappy, or do something destructive. That's because they simply don't know that men have the same sort of stress response to cortisol chaos as women do. If they've been taught to just suck it up and deal with it, they push the truth further away, making everything worse.

Men, just like women, need a hormone plan. They should also be tracking their hormone levels, and this means establishing a good relationship with a medical provider who is focused on optimization and vitality and not just on preventing disease. Now, to get them to that appointment—that's a whole different book.

Dealing with Anxiety

If I had to pick the dominant emotion for Superwomen, it would be anxiety.

This is a phase during which so many symptoms of anxiety—heart palpitations, sweaty repetitive thoughts, that disconnected floating-out-of-body feeling—can take over. Often, this anxiety is physically rooted, especially when you don't yet have control over how your body is changing. Anticipating a hot flash or an episode of brain fog when you've got important duties at work or at home can leave any woman a bundle of nerves.

There are also emotional triggers of anxiety. There could be anxiety about having a baby or not having had one yet, or not having met the right partner to father that baby—rooted in fears the fertility window is closing. For women who do have families, there's anxiety about how they look and feel and, often, concern about their status with regard to their partner. In fact, I see relationship anxiety with startling frequency in my Superwomen patients. Sometimes these couples have been together for a while, in a comfortable but boring groove, and they start thinking, *Wait a minute, I'm getting older and I haven't done XYZ yet, so I need that opportunity*. Or, if their relationship is struggling, they may feel it's safer to cling to something that's not healthy rather than face an unknown outcome. These emotional triggers and stress create more anxiety, fear, and trauma for the body, which then responds with hormone disruption. Chinese medicine predicts this: fear and anxiety are stored in the liver, and the liver is responsible for managing and packaging the hormones. It's no surprise that your hormones go haywire at this stage—which is why it's so important to get them under control.

Those "Time's Running Out" and "Living on Borrowed Time" Feelings

Time is a huge commodity for Superwomen. The kids, the career, the parents, the unpredictable perimenopause symptoms. It's even harder for the sandwich generation, or women who have to manage the stress of child-rearing while also taking care of aging parents.

I see a lot of sadness and grief in Superwomen, owing to whatever is going on in their personal lives—and their sense of loss of youth or time. Even as I head into my fifties, I still have a little bit of that broody urge and wonder if I should have had one more child. It's that time-is-running-out feeling.

Or, maybe your life choices were upended unexpectedly, as happened to one of my patients. She came to me when she was in her mid-forties and had been married for fifteen years. Her husband never wanted children and so she had multiple abortions. Now, the relationship was falling apart and she was filled with grief because she'd put his choices ahead of her own. "I don't know why I listened to him," she said as she sat sobbing in my office. "And now not only will I not have my relationship, but I also won't have children. I won't be able to have a family." My heart was breaking for her.

Your chemistry, biology, and physiology determine your bandwidth, or your emotional and mental capacity to do something. They determine the choices you make in life, from what you eat and drink to how you feel and think. And balancing your hormones is a part of that story. The Thirty-Day Hormone Reset (Chapter 9) presented in this book will help you do exactly that. Hormone symptoms can be subtle—until they are a big problem. Don't wait for something to be completely obvious before you check it out.

Where Did My Libido Go?

Sexual behavior as you get older is one of those topics my patients want to avoid. Some of them are embarrassed or ashamed that they've gained weight or are unhappy in their bodies. They don't feel sexy because they think they don't look sexy (even if they still do!). And it is true that when the female hormone levels decline, libido can decline with them, along with vaginal lubrication and the ability to orgasm.

I don't believe that low or nonexistent libido is healthy. If anything, Superwomen should be coming into their sexual prowess. If you think back to the dynamics of sexuality in your twenties, you usually remember trying to please your partner; in your thirties and forties, you might have been a fertility machine, having babies and breastfeeding and raising children. Then you are done with all that by your fifties and you can actually maybe enjoy it? Sex is now finally about you and your partner.

Sadly, that's often not what happens. When your hormones drop, this lends itself to a feeling of being expired. You will *not* feel expired if you're having regular orgasms, however. If you aren't having sex owing to low libido, this can be addressed in the exam room—first, by checking for hormone imbalances, and then by addressing the emotional part.

Who wants to spend the rest of their life not having sex? It's definitely a vital sign for a relationship, not just as an expression of love and desire for your partner but also in terms of your energy centers functioning optimally. I've experienced this personally, as my sex drive can dwindle when I'm exhausted, and then I shut down. We don't realize the *consequences* of that shutting down, though. So, when my patients tell me their libido has vanished, we dig deeper to find the cause. Of course, if they are oblivious to the topic and the conversation, I don't push it—although I do tell them that a healthy sexual appetite is an important sign of energy and vitality.

How Hormonal Shifts Affect Your Face

I often hear concern from Superwomen about their skin. Lower estrogen levels affect the collagen and elastin levels, so the skin isn't as vibrant and smooth as it used to be. Skin-cell turnover slows with age, so you might look more blah. If there's any toxicity in your body, your skin often is the first place where it shows. And despite lavish claims by skin-care companies, topical products can do only so much. This can lead to a panic response, in which Superwomen run to procedures before they think it will be too late to do any good.

Let me say right now that I'm not against aesthetic procedures. There are options for altering your appearance that didn't exist even a few scant years ago. When it comes to hair, for example, problems arise commonly during perimenopause, and they can be incredibly upsetting because hair is such a visible sign of aging. Hormonal decline means the grays start to appear, the hair texture changes, and thinning can become noticeable.

But here's the problem: If you don't fix the inside first, and you keep searching for that procedure you think is going to make you feel better on the outside, that procedure is unlikely to work as well as it is meant to. If, for example, you're losing estrogen, that explains why your skin is sagging. If you're losing progesterone, that is why you're not sleeping and you are gaining more wrinkles. If you have a lot of inflammation, any exfoliating or laser treatments won't be as effective as they could be. Lots of women run to do PRP (platelet-rich plasma) for hair loss, but it won't work if their hormones are imbalanced, as the hair follicles won't be activated.

In other words, your aesthetic journey should be secondary to the chemistry of your internal hormone journey. But in our society, it's the other way around. The end result is a lot of wasted money and energy as well as women who are unhappy with their treatments. Let me repeat: you need to get your hormones back on track *first*.

Also, Superstars often feel bad about themselves or think some aspect of their appearance looks bad because they themselves are in a bad place. For instance, my husband always knows when I'm about to start my period, because three days before my cycle, I will invariably say, "I hate my hair, I hate this, I hate that." Then I get my period and I'm like, "Oh my god, my hair is great! Look how thick it is now!"

The whole point of fixing your hormones in your forties is to gain an internal glow. When you're healthy on the inside, you're always going to look better on the outside. Hormone balancing may be the ultimate beauty secret.

Not Expired, but Rewired

The clarion call of this hormone phase is to rewire. You rewire your thoughts, your actions, and your journey to be the person you want to be: the Journey UP. It's the call to heal prior wounds, the call to release your anger and baggage—physically and energetically—so you can move on to what's next. Not to see perimenopause as a stopping point; rather, to see it as a spiritual starting point.

Forty is a turning point. Forty is when you need to know the foods that are right for you, or else your metabolism will revolt. You need to sleep deeply, or your hormones will shift. You need balance and challenge in your career and in your personal life, or your body will tell you. You can't just hide from your issues; you need to be in the right place. Because when you're in harmony with your body and with what your body needs, you'll find that the Superwoman years can be the best ever.

To me, women in their forties look better than they've ever looked before. I think she was exaggerating, but somebody told me the other day that she couldn't believe I was turning fifty, that she thought I was thirty! Now, I know I don't *look* thirty (just compare my pics), but I sure *feel* thirty because I have my personal health recipe. And this is what I want to create for you.

If, on the other hand, you've been ignoring all those warning signs about your health and your hormones, turning forty might not feel like a celebration. It's time to dump the baggage and get rewired. When you don't believe you've got so much vibrant life ahead of you, it's awfully hard to look up. But this can change, and I will show you how.

As you gallop into the final years of the Superwoman phase, I want to see you being your authentic self. The responsibilities of childrearing and family relationships should be easing, and as the pressure starts to lower, there's opportunity for more creativity, mentorship, and leadership. This is your spiritual and energetic starting point—your journey back to *you*.

No more excuses. I can't tell you how many times I've heard the excuse "I've just got to take care of this one or that one, and nobody can do it but me. I'll deal with my own stuff later." Sometimes that is unavoidable reality, but if it's just an excuse for you not to come into your potential, it's time to change that internal dialogue and develop a plan that leads you to decisions that serve your highest purpose. And that's exactly what we are going to do here together, in my Thirty-Day Hormone Reset (Chapter 9).

It's showtime. It's time to flip the page, make changes in your life, and increase your bandwidth. You've earned the right to be the star. The curtains are rising very soon. Let's go. Time to show the world your stuff.

The Superwoman's Top Three Checklist

1. If you feel that you are just getting old, pause the negative thinking and get your hormone levels checked (see page 124).
2. If your perimenopause symptoms become debilitating, start building a team of hormone doctors and nutritionists who can help you put the pieces of your hormone puzzle together.

3. Step into your purpose. Consider what may be blocking you; for example, write in a journal for ten minutes daily for six weeks. That can help you outline and fine-tune your desires while also releasing your frustrations. In your journal, make a Joy List and a Hate List. Remove items from the Hate List and add ones to the Joy List. (We will do more of this work in Chapter 9.)

5. The Commander Shift: Taking Charge

Age 56+

Key Word: Depression

The Commanders are what I call the women in this amazing age group—gifted in knowledge, strength, resilience, and so much more.

By now, you are well aware of the superpowers you already possess. You know your strengths, weaknesses, and how to eat for energy, and you have a personalized body map to wellness—at least I hope you do. And if you don't, we will create one. As you move forward, the goal is to stay in command and bring your gifts and superpowers to those around you.

These years bring us back full circle to where we started this conversation: with hormones and hormonal health in adolescence. Some women benefit from continued hormone replacement; others don't seem to need or want it. But *all* women need to stay on top of matters concerning their gut and liver health. These organs are our primary means of detoxification; they need to function properly to filter out toxins, environmental pollutants, hormone metabolites, and other chemicals that cause inflammation and disease. And, yes, their functioning does slow down as we get older (notice I did not say *age*).

Hormonal Decline Is Real—But You Can Do Something About It

At this stage of life there is continued decline in metabolism and hormone levels—we can't lie about that. Some or all of your perimenopause symptoms might continue, thanks to lower levels of estrogen, progesterone, and testosterone. You might have issues with bone density, hot flashes, lower energy, cholesterol levels, disrupted sleep, moodiness, skin, and hair. And there's no magic pill that will reverse this process. But there are many things you can do to slow the process down, reduce the symptoms, have more energy, and feel more vibrant.

Most women at this point have gone through menopause, which is clinically defined as having no periods for one year. This most commonly takes places when a woman is in her late forties; the average age in the United States is fifty-two. Menopause used to be called the "change of life." And it is a change, but it's one where women finally gain knowledge of themselves—they understand their health needs, their hormone map, how emotions impact their body, and how they guide their decisions.

It Can Be Very Hard Not to Get Depressed

One of the reasons I named this age group the Commanders is that they have done IT—they have been there, done that. They have weathered disappointments and enjoyed successes, felt joys and suffered losses. This can be an illness-free, low-medication period of time, or it can be one during which women can get seriously ill, thanks to that unavoidable intersection of environment, life and lifestyle choices, and genetics, all of which are at play.

Many of the women I see are fearful that they are going to need a lot of medication and more intensive treatments for their hormonal issues. They are worried they are going to get sick or that something's wrong now, which is a legitimate concern. This fear can be exacerbated by our traditional medical system, which doesn't allow practitioners to think outside the box. Hence, physicians downplay your symptoms, having been taught that aging is normal and does not need intervention. And if you've spent a lifetime not being able to speak up or question your doctors or the system, it only gets harder with each passing year.

For some Commanders, depression can seep in, creating further roadblocks to feeling good. There are biochemical reasons, with lower hormone levels and a less efficient processing of the nutrients needed for normal amounts of brain chemicals. But there are also deeply emotional reasons for depression, as loved ones may get sick, children leave the nest, and relationships and community support systems may begin to shift. Retirement may also force Commanders to leave behind a built-in support system and the safety of a consistent schedule. It's not surprising that depression may set in.

Depression can creep into your world over time, so you don't realize quite how bad you feel until you feel terrible. Depression leads to poor choices, which then worsen the key health concepts that lead to disease: inflammation, nutritional deficiencies, increased toxic load, and mitochondrial dysfunction.

Signs of Depression

According to the National Institutes of Health, you may be depressed if any of these symptoms persist for at least two weeks:

- Persistent sad, anxious, or "empty" mood
- Feelings of hopelessness or pessimism

- Irritability
- Feelings of guilt, worthlessness, or helplessness
- Decreased energy or fatigue
- Difficulty sleeping, early morning awakening, or oversleeping
- Loss of interest or pleasure in hobbies and activities
- Moving or talking more slowly
- Feeling restless or having trouble sitting still
- Difficulty concentrating, remembering, or making decisions
- Changes in appetite or weight
- Thoughts of death or suicide, or suicide attempts
- Aches or pains, headaches, cramps, or digestive problems without a clear physical cause that do not ease even with treatment

How do we snap Commanders out of depression? That is the magic question. I saw depression in my mother-in-law, I can see it in my mom, and I see it in my Commander patients—a slow, insidious low-grade malaise that they have trouble articulating to me.

But it does not have to be this way.

When it comes to aging, women have a decision to make. You can age like Jane Fonda or Jane Seymour or Susan Lucci, who are all seventy-plus and *amazingly* youthful. Or, you can give up. I have patients who have done just that. They're still relatively healthy physically, but there's a sort of droop to them. They are clinically depressed even if they don't want to admit it. Their mantra is *I'm old, I'm done.* They ask themselves, *What should I do now? I don't look good anymore. Nothing I do matters. Do I have any worth? Do I have any purpose?*

My mother-in-law felt that way. She didn't think she was capable enough to learn a new skill, or take on a new hobby, or meet new people. My husband and I tried to help her as best we could, but we were so sad that she was always so lonely, yet she was never able to shift her thinking.

I think the biggest gift Commanders can give themselves is to let go of their fears and their tendency to cling to what they know. That clinging to the familiar so hampers their personal growth and their ability to enjoy who and where they are *right now*. When you don't feel good, you're not willing to take risks. For example, if you've always wanted to sing, now is the time to join the chorus. If you've always wanted to travel to Antarctica, now's the time to book that trip. Taking risks and putting yourself out there leads to this phase of life as exciting, rather than as a concluding chapter—it's the *best* life, not the change of life.

If, however, you aren't getting better and you remain depressed, please seek professional help. There are many treatment options for depression, including herbs, supplements, and acupuncture, in addition to counseling, support groups, and therapy. A good therapist who will listen well can be a lifesaver. It is a tough place to be in, as many people who haven't suffered from depression sometimes offer unsolicited and unhelpful advice that can make you feel even worse. You might be prescribed antidepressants, which can work well or might have side effects; you won't know, though, until you try a medication, as results can't be predicted. I know of women in their nineties who were prescribed antidepressants for the first time in their lives, and they were astounded by how much better they felt. You're never too old to seek treatment for any mental health issue.

For our Commanders, time is now a commodity. You know how important it is to make your time count, to age gracefully and with vitality. It's a moment when you sit and look in the mirror, and you define what aging particularly means to you. Does that necessarily mean you want to look and feel thirty again? Or, does that mean you want to have the energy to get up, go on with your day, sleep through the night, maintain your muscle mass, be sharp and focused, and be able to participate in family and community events? To be that respected mentor people turn to for advice because you've *lived it*? This is, after all, often a time when people run for political office, or dig into nonprofit and charitable work, or spend as much time as they can with their grandchildren. These are all important roles that Commanders should not be running away from. Younger generations might have more hormones, but you have more wisdom. It's up to you to be confident enough to use that wisdom to continue to thrive.

The Commander's Top Three Checklist

1. Get full medical checkups twice a year, with blood work done to check all your hormone levels (see page 124). If you have any new hormonally related symptoms, get them checked out by specialists, if needed.
2. Resist sliding into depression. There are answers out there, from food choices to medicines to hormones, and everything in between, that can improve your emotional state.
3. Let go of your fears and enjoy who and where you are, right now. You're a Commander, and don't you forget it!

chapter 2

The Signs of a Shift

Symptoms of Hormone Imbalance

Hormonal imbalances are insidious, with the individual hormone levels shifting slowly, leading to symptoms you may not notice right away. Having trouble sleeping? Well, of course; you've been extra stressed out by a huge project at work. Skin breaking out and a few extra pounds creeping on? No surprise; you've been eating more junk food for comfort lately because you just broke up with your boyfriend. Feeling extra cranky? That's because the bills are piling up and the car needs new tires. You knuckle down and try to push through it.

But no matter the cause, it's *how you feel* that matters. You probably don't even care whether I diagnose the situation as a hormone imbalance or an alien disease from outer space—you just want to feel better, feel stronger, and be like yourself again. Here's the good news about hormone imbalances (unlike alien diseases from outer space): we can get you feeling better by rebalancing those hormones and managing your symptoms.

So now, let's take a look at some of the most common hormone symptoms I see in my practices at CentreSpringMD. We won't be getting into solutions just yet, but that information is in the next few chapters. You'll take the knowledge you gain here with you into the next chapters, and you will better understand why the merging of Eastern and Western medicine works so well to balance your hormones.

You can come back to this chapter to check in with yourself maybe every few months. Remember, we as women are fluid, cyclical creatures. What works today may not work tomorrow. Your symptoms can change over time.

Here is my comprehensive Hormone Symptom Checklist. Go ahead and take a minute to mark which symptoms you may be suffering from right now.

The Hormone Symptom Checklist

Symptom	Yes	No
Acne		
ADHD		
Anxiety		
Belly fat		
Bloating		
Burning tongue		
Brain fog		
Cold intolerance		
Constipation		

Symptom	Yes	No
Depression		
Diarrhea		
Facial hair		
Fatigue		
Hair loss		
Heavy periods		
Hot flashes		
IBS		
Irregular periods		
Insomnia		
Joint pain		
Joint swelling		
Low libido		
Night sweats		
Painful periods		
Palpitations		
Reflux		
Sweating		
Weight gain		
Weight loss		
Vaginal discharge		
Vaginal dryness		
Yeast infections		

If you checked more than five of these symptoms, it's likely you have a hormone imbalance and are in Hormone Hell. What you might not realize is that your body is no stranger to these imbalances; they've been happening throughout your life. You need to understand *which* hormones are imbalanced and *which* are causing your symptoms so you can follow the best course of treatment.

Thankfully, after years of experience working with women and their hormones, I've detected various patterns. Here are the symptoms I keep seeing over and over again.

Rock Star (Ages 13–19)

Condition	Hormones to Check
Acne	DHT, testosterone, free testosterone, DHEAs
Anxiety	Progesterone, TSH, total and free T4/T3
Bloating	Estrogen, progesterone
Cramps/pain (with period)	Estrogen, progesterone
Depression	Methyl B$_{12}$, methyl folate, progesterone, estradiol, estrone
Irregular periods	Progesterone, insulin, total and free testosterone, estradiol, estrone

Hustler (Ages 20–28)

Symptom	Hormones/Conditions to Check
Acne	High testosterone, DHT, DHEAs, androgens
Fatigue	Adrenal fatigue/thyroid imbalances
Hair loss	High testosterone, DHT, androgens
Mid-cycle spotting	High estradiol, estrone, fibroids
Joint pain	Low progesterone, *Candida*, food intolerances
Painful periods	High estradiol, estrone, low progesterone, ovarian cysts, endometriosis
Rectal pain	Endometriosis
Weight gain	High estradiol, estrone, insulin

Superstar (Ages 29–38)

Symptom	Hormones/Conditions to Check
Wired but tired (up all night and tired all day), with disrupted sleep, focus, and energy, more anxiety and depression, signs of inflammation, joint pain, memory loss, or just chronic fatigue	Cortisol, adrenaline
Breast tenderness, mid-cycle spotting, migraines, endometriosis, weight gain, depression	Estrogen dominance (high estrone, stored estrogen)
Acne, hair loss, irregular cycles, insulin resistance	High androgens (testosterone, DHT, free testosterone and DHEAs)
Belly fat, weight gain, back fat	Insulin resistance
Hair loss, weight gain, constipation, infertility, joint pain, heavy periods, estrogen dominance	Thyroid instability

Superwoman (Ages 39–55)

Symptom/Condition	Hormones/Conditions to Check
Anxiety	Low progesterone, high or low cortisol
Brain fog	Low progesterone, pregenalone, estradiol
Constipation	Low magnesium, thyroid instability, high estradiol, high estrone
Depression	High or low estrogen, thyroid imbalance
Fatigue	Adrenal fatigue, thyroid imbalance, low iron, low B vitamins, low vitamin D
Hair loss	Thyroid instability, high androgens, high DHT
Inflammation	Low progesterone, *Candida*, bacterial overgrowth
Insomnia	Low progesterone, low estrogen
Joint pain	Low progesterone, high estradiol
Skin issues (acne, psoriasis)	High androgens
Weight gain	Insulin resistance, estrogen dominance, thyroid instability

Commander (Ages 55+)

Condition	Hormones/Patterns to Check
Bone health	Leaky gut, thyroid imbalance, low estradiol, progesterone, insulin
Cancer prevention	Liver sluggishness, mitochondrial dysfunction, inflammation
Cognitive decline/brain fog	Low progesterone, estradiol, vitamins D and B
Gut heath	*Candida*, fat malabsorption, pancreatic insufficiency
Heart health	Low estradiol, high insulin, leaky gut
Inflammation	Leaky gut/low omega-3/low vitamin D/hormone depletion/high insulin
Joint pain/musculoskeletal	Leaky gut/low estradiol, low progesterone, high insulin
Weight gain	Insulin resistance, estrogen dominance, thyroid instability

The Common Symptoms of Hormone Imbalance

There are symptoms (how you feel), and then there are actual diagnoses or conditions (what they are called or labeled). You may have heard these labels in your doctor visits, but they are not often used in connection with your hormones or to describe a hormone pattern. Your instinct might be to look for quick remedies for each symptom you're experiencing, but in my practice I look for the *root cause* of the symptoms, and I aim to heal the whole body rather than applying quick-fix solutions to individual symptoms. When we get to the Thirty-Day Hormone Reset, we address ways to balance your hormones and alleviate these symptoms. But for now, let's commit to just learning the basics. Remember, knowledge is power.

Ready? Here we go. . . .

Acne

A condition that affected me personally, acne is not just about puberty and junk food. It is, in actuality, a full expression of skin inflammation; that is, the skin is rebelling against the body's chemistry by telling you it's not happy.

Acne is caused by a bacterium that is always found on your skin, called *Propionibacterium acnes*, or *P. acnes* for short. Usually, that bacterium is balanced by other bacteria to keep it in check, but under the right conditions (excess oil that clogs pores, a buildup of the dead skin cells in the topmost layer of your epidermis, a shift in your gut microbiome, and, of course, an overproduction of certain hormones) *P. acnes* can grow and spread, causing breakouts. The jaw, chin, and neck breakouts are most often connected to high androgen levels, while the forehead and cheek breakouts are often more gut based—usually alterations in the microbiome and inflammation that then trigger an inflammatory response. Acne can be devastating for teens and just as devastating for women (and men) of all ages who suddenly start having the condition or have a recurrence just when they thought it was gone for good.

When we apply the EastWest approach to a condition like acne, we know that the gut, hormones, stress, diet, and sleep patterns all influence this confidence-killing skin issue. But there are answers—without heavy medications—when we focus primarily on balancing the gut and the hormones to achieve healthy skin.

Brain Fog

I was a classic go-getter: I climbed the corporate ladder quickly and was soon in charge of human resources for a billion-dollar company. My CEO could depend on me; he'd call me at any time and I'd have the answers at my fingertips . . . until I slowly noticed embarrassing changes. When questioned about a potential hire, I mixed up the names and résumés, leading to almost hiring the wrong executive for a particular role. I started forgetting thoughts mid-sentence; and while I thought no one noticed, as I struggled to keep it together, my CEO called me in to find out what was wrong. I was mortified and I realized I needed help fast, or I would surely soon be out of a job.

—Sara King, age 51

Ever feel overwhelmed by your to-do list and not sure where to start? It happens to all of us. So many of my patients describe going from go-getter and multitasker (Hustler/Superwoman prototypes) to being unable to remember names, give a presentation, or find their purse.

Hormonal brain fog tends to be more gradual, but then it becomes chronic. There's a distinct change along the lines of *I used to be able to do all this stuff, and now it's taking me twice as long to get through a task that used to take fifteen minutes.* The influence of hormones on your brain is noticeable in all women, from Rock Stars to Commanders. I work with a lot of adolescents who have attention and focus issues—oftentimes they have ADHD triggered by crazy hormones. Hormone issues can really affect your brainpower.

Specifically, progesterone, insulin, estrogen, the thyroid hormones, and even the androgens are usually the culprits behind brain fog. Progesterone and pregnenalone are notorious for causing cognitive deficits. The brain fog associated with low progesterone is steady, leading to a loss of words and the names of things. On the other hand, the brain fog associated with high estrogen almost bleeds into depression; in certain populations, it can be the kick-starter of dementia. Insulin triggers cognitive issues that seem to be on a roller coaster, up and down like the rising and falling levels of blood sugar in the body. Whatever situation you might have, brain fog can be particularly frustrating when it affects your ability to do your work effectively. And it can even be dangerous if your mind wanders when you're driving, operating machinery, or caring for others.

But brain fog can be lifted. We just need to get your hormones balanced.

Diabetes

Diabetes is a metabolic disease that is either *genetic*, meaning there is an existing predisposition, or *behavioral*, meaning that lifestyle factors contributed to the expression of the disease. Shockingly, nearly 26 million children and adults in the United States have diabetes, and another 79 million Americans have pre-diabetic conditions and are at risk for developing Type 2 diabetes. Diabetes is a chronic disease that can't be ignored, as it can lead to nerve damage, blindness, kidney failure, cardiovascular disease, and early death.

The Five Types of Diabetes

Insulin is a hormone produced in the pancreas that helps the cells absorb and metabolize blood sugar, or glucose, and gives these cells the energy they need to function properly. Without enough insulin, or if the cells can't process it properly, the glucose builds up in the blood and eventually becomes stored in the body as fat.

TYPE 1: This is a genetic condition in which the cells in the pancreas are attacked and become unable to make enough insulin to push the blood sugar where it needs to go. It is an autoimmune disease, and the symptoms are progressive if it's not managed with daily injections of insulin, as well as diet and lifestyle management.

TYPE 1.5: This type of diabetes is similar to Type 1, but it presents later in life and is also an autoimmune disease or disease of inflammation. The body develops antibodies to the pancreas, resulting in decreased insulin production and high blood sugar. Many of the symptoms of hyperglycemia can present as sweating, dizziness, excessive thirst, and excessive urination.

TYPE 2: This form of diabetes is associated with excessive weight, food consumption, and insulin resistance. Insulin resistance occurs when the pancreas cannot keep up with the demand of insulin needs; this in turn leads to more glucose floating around in the bloodstream. The muscle, fat, and liver cells don't respond to the higher levels of insulin and blood sugar, causing more fat storage and the release of even more insulin. Eventually the pancreas cannot keep up with the demand for insulin, glucose levels rise, you feel hungry even if you just ate so you eat some more—causing another insulin spike. It's a vicious cycle that can be hard to reverse.

TYPE 3: Alzheimer's disease is now being referred to as Type 3 diabetes. Yes, the most recent research finds that it is an insulin-based disease rather than a brain-based disease, because the chronic inflammation caused by insulin resistance triggers neuro-inflammation and dementia.

TYPE 4: Technically, there is no Type 4, but some people are batting around this term as a form of insulin resistance in the elderly. These people aren't overweight or obese, and they don't necessarily have pancreatic issues. But they're losing so much skeletal muscle—and muscle is actually an important endocrine organ. Muscle mass has been shown in research to improve the movement of glucose from the bloodstream into the cells, increasing insulin sensitivity. In fact, a recent study has shown that for every 10 percent increase in skeletal muscle to body weight, there is an 11 percent reduction in the risk of insulin resistance and a 12 percent drop in the risk of pre-diabetes. Still don't like the gym? I had to get over it, too. . . .

NON-DIABETIC HYPOGLYCEMIA: This condition is one in which blood sugar drops below 55 μg/dl, but without accompanying diabetes. This can be caused by dietary, lifestyle, illness, medications, or genetic factors. Tracking the blood sugars is often helpful in this scenario to help diagnose and manage blood sugars and keep the insulin balanced.

Endometriosis

One of the most devastating and painful hormonal conditions is endometriosis, which happens when the lining of the inside of the uterus (the endometrium) grows outside of the uterus rather than inside, where it belongs. This tissue can then appear most commonly in the abdomen—in the ovaries, intestines, fallopian tubes, or peritoneal cavity. Worse, endometrial tissue on the outside of the uterus responds to the same hormones as it does when it's on the inside. Thus, it responds to the menstrual cycle and bleeds. This leads to inflammation, as well as scar tissue, adhesions, cysts, and most of all, excruciating pain.

Unfortunately, only a biopsy or surgery can accurately diagnose endometriosis. Lab tests, CT scans, or ultrasounds can't confirm it, so many women who suffer from it are not treated properly and/or are misdiagnosed. I meet so many frustrated women who ultimately get this diagnosis but have had life-long hormone imbalances that were never addressed. In fact, it takes on average eight years after the onset of symptoms for most women to receive the right treatment or diagnosis. Instead, they're told to take painkillers or to go on hormonal birth control, which may slightly mitigate symptoms but not treat the problem itself. Surgery can, however, remove the excess tissue.

It is possible, however, through lab testing and ultrasound, to understand your risks for endometriosis. Understanding your hormone levels and how your body uses hormones can lead to an earlier diagnosis.

Fibroids

Fibroids are growths of the uterus that are usually non-cancerous and appear most frequently in in women in their twenties and thirties. These growths, also known as myomas or leiomyomas, can continue to grow and stay present until women reach menopause. For many women, fibroids become a source of severe menstrual pain, heavy bleeding, and anemia. I see fibroids more often in women of color, and there are some studies that indicate there may be a connection between fibroids and chemical hair relaxers.

Conventionally, fibroids are usually a watch-and-wait diagnosis, but as they get larger they can impact fertility, gut health, and overall energy. For these reasons, many women have to get their fibroids taken out, a procedure known as a myomectomy, or end up getting their uterus removed (hysterectomy) when they are done having children.

Again, this could all be prevented. There is a gut-liver-hormone connection when it comes to fibroids, which could be discovered if we all started having more detailed hormone evaluations.

Fatigue

I've traveled the world, thanks to my high-powered career in sales, and I now live on a farm, having taken an early retirement. But I'm exhausted; when I should be enjoying the fruits of my labor, I can't get out of bed and get going with my day. In fact, the distance from my bed to the door to start the day is overwhelming, making me dread even the fun stuff like walking or seeing a friend.

—*Patricia Short, age 43*

Why are we so exhausted? Is it from multitasking all day long or is it our hormones? Or is it both? When you have regular fatigue, you can go get a massage, or work out, or have dinner with your partner or your girlfriends and you soon feel better. You were just super-tired and you didn't sleep well because you were going over that presentation you had to give at work, but once it was over, you knew you'd be able to recharge. There's a solution: if you're able to break free of the stress-and-overwhelm cycle, then your energy is better, your mood is more stable, and it's easier to lose weight.

When your fatigue is hormone-based, however, you do all those stress-busting or energizing activities that usually work—but there's no moving the needle. It's almost like you're walking through knee-high mud. That's when so many of my patients break down crying in my office, because they still feel like crap, even though they are making life changes—they're eating healthily, they're going to acupuncture, they have a bedtime routine.

When I hear that, my diagnosis of a hormonal issue can be easier to present to them. I explain that if I describe hormonal fatigue symptoms to a practitioner of Chinese medicine, they will say, "We're so tired because our livers are sick of us and have given up, and it's show-ing in our hormones." And further, I explain that we're all pushing ourselves to the max, whether we are raising children or building busi-nesses or whatever else we're doing; we're in the center of everything and our livers are fed up with our cortisol levels going higher and higher and higher . . . until they crash.

That is the reason why so many of us are beyond exhaustion. Our bodies are in a state of chronic inflammation and liver toxicity, causing hormone disruption. Our immune systems are shot. We're vulnerable to every bug that's out there. We just don't know when to say no. It's part of Superwoman syndrome—of not knowing how to identify our boundaries, how to nurture ourselves, how to dial it all back. It's be-cause that kind of behavior is often not rewarded, and we don't know how to honor ourselves. When were you rewarded last time for sleep-ing eight hours? Who said, "Good job! Wow, eight full and uninter-rupted hours! I'm so proud of you!"

My guess is no one has ever said that to you. And if someone did say it, I bet you felt guilty about accepting the honor. Now, it's time to get balanced. Get hormone balanced, life balanced, and liver balanced. I'll take bets that your Hormone Symptom Checklist (page 62) will shrink.

Irritable Bowel/Bloating/Constipation

I go the bathroom regularly every day. I don't have acid reflux. I don't have a lot of gas. Why are you talking about my gut?

—Tanisha Washington, age 36

I get asked this question a lot. Your gut health is not just about diges-tion; it's ground zero for your health. It's the foundation of your entire house and the source of your hormone superpower.

Hormonal imbalances and gut dysfunction go together, so this is a central concept when approaching hormone balancing the holistic EastWest way. When your gut is not working well, you can't get the nutrients from the healthy foods you are eating, your gut bacteria goes out of balance, and your gut cannot package the hormones to go where they need to go—to the bloodstream for activity and to the liver for detoxification. Hormone imbalances also impact the gut. Progesterone deficiency can cause *Candida* overgrowth, a fungal infection; too much estrogen can cause bloating, constipation, diarrhea, and an overactive thyroid.

The gut–hormone connections are fundamental in Eastern systems of medicine, and they are a fine starting point for treating hormone imbalances.

Hair Loss/Excess Hair

I'm almost afraid to brush my hair anymore because the amount of hair I see in the brush really scares me. I haven't changed any of my hair products. But my hair loss is starting to be visible and I don't know what to do.

—*Reena Patel, age 34*

Your menstrual cycle is a vital sign, your hormones are a vital sign, and your hair is a vital sign, too; loss of hair or too much hair is often the result of hormone imbalances. For instance, too much facial or body hair signifies high androgens and testosterone. Without enough of the thyroid hormones T4 and T3, or an imbalance in the pituitary hormone TSH, individual hair follicles don't have the support they need to grow, making your hair thinner or sparser all over the scalp. Declining levels of estrogen and progesterone during perimenopause and menopause also trigger hair loss. High androgens or male hormones result in hair becoming drier, more brittle, and wiry, and then eventually falling out. This resultant hair loss is called *androgenetic alopecia*, and it is common in PCOS, or polycystic ovarian syndrome.

Pregnancy is also responsible for changes in hair. Many women are thrilled when their hair becomes thicker and more lush during the nine months of pregnancy, but they are devastated when their glorious tresses suddenly begin to fall out after the baby is born. That's because pregnancy alters your hair's normal growth cycle, preventing it from shedding. When the estrogen and other hormones decrease rapidly postpartum, along with changes in metabolism and the likely stress of caring for a newborn during sleepless nights, the hair will start to be shed. Usually, though, your hair returns to normal after six months.

In practice, I try to identify the following hair-loss patterns:

- Thyroid-based hair loss is often most noticeable at the scalp and falls out easily—literally, with one brush-through with your hand, hair is everywhere—but the texture remains the same.
- Androgen-mediated or male-pattern hair loss results in the hair first becoming paper thin and wiry, then falling out.
- Estrogen and progesterone-based hair loss appears at the temples.
- Nutritionally based hair loss leads to brittle and dry hair that grays, easily breaks, and does not grow.

Hot Flashes/Night Sweats

I can't stand myself. I keep gaining weight, I can't make good choices to save my life, and the biggest problem is that I'm not

sleeping. I've been having hot flashes and night sweats for years—
and I wake up exhausted every morning. Because I'm so tired,
sugar, caffeine, and nightly drinks have become my constant
companions. I need them to help me get through the day of tasks
and responsibilities at hand.

—Renata Sims, age 53

Hot flashes and night sweats are two of the most visible signs of a hormonal imbalance, especially in perimenopause; it's definitely an Achilles' heel for most women. These symptoms are caused by fluctuations in your estrogen levels—sometimes high and sometimes low—leaving you tired, wired, foggy, or irritable. But there are solutions for hot flashes and night sweats, and many of these solutions begin with establishing a healthy gut, liver, and clean diet. Gentle hormone balancing may also relieve these symptoms.

Incontinence

I can't remember the last time I had an uninterrupted night's sleep,
because I am always waking up to pee. Sometimes the urge comes
when I've only been in bed for a few minutes and I shouldn't have
to go—but then I do!

—Grace Liu, age 38

Do you have to suddenly run to the bathroom when you only just went? Do you feel a desperate urge to pee but then not a whole lot comes out? Hormone shifts can leave you incontinent and with a sense of urgency that you simply cannot hold your bladder. Low progesterone and estrogen are the most common causes of this symptom—and can be corrected.

Infertility

A woman who's been trying for a baby with no success after a year is considered infertile. This is one of the most difficult situations women longing to be mothers can face, and it is also more common than many people realize. According to the Centers for Disease Control, "in the United States, among heterosexual women aged fifteen to forty-nine years with no prior births, about one in five (19 percent) are unable to get pregnant after one year of trying. One in four (26 percent) women in this group have difficulty getting pregnant or carrying a pregnancy to term (impaired fecundity)."

There are many potential causes of infertility, and hormonal conditions are among them. These conditions can include PCOS, thyroid disorders, endometriosis, fibroids, undiagnosed diabetes, or insulin resistance, or structural issues with the fallopian tubes. High levels of stress that lead to elevated cortisol levels can block ovulation, which is essential for pregnancy. Globally, male sperm counts are also declining, making fertility a seemingly elusive challenge.

Irregular and Heavy Menstrual Cycles

When I stood up, blood was running down my legs, staining the chair and my clothes. I was horrified. It looked like a bad horror film. I cannot live like this—just take this uterus out of me already, please!

—Ashley Grogam, age 48

Since progesterone regulates the second half of the menstrual cycle, you need it to shed the uterine lining. With lower levels of progesterone, though, the estrogen becomes more dominant and you're not able to fully shed the lining every month, which then intensifies the flow in your next cycle. Your periods can become super-heavy and super-painful. My patients tell me that they are bleeding through their underwear and they are afraid to go anywhere away from home.

There are many causes of irregular and heavy period cycles, including low progesterone, an imbalanced thyroid, high insulin, and high or low cortisol. Again, the hormones work in concert—and heavy cycles don't have one singular cause.

Joint Pain and Bone Health

One of the most fascinating observations gained from my practice is that hormone shifts trigger flares or expressions of autoimmune syndromes. Many women come in with new-onset joint pain or joint swelling, and as we run the diagnostics, we find that they may have previously undetected rheumatoid arthritis, Sjögren syndrome, or even "gray zone" inflammation, something that does not get a true diagnosis or a label but is in actuality an autoimmune syndrome.

Joint Pain

Inflammation is what drives a lot of pain, but it is usually not associated with hormone shifts. When faced with inflammation, most folks think they simply worked out too hard or did not stretch enough. In many cases, though, hormones play a role in the inflammatory cycle.

Progesterone, for example, is an anti-inflammatory hormone. Many autoimmune diseases flare up when there are downward shifts in progesterone. Thyroid imbalances and high insulin levels will also influence inflammation. Correcting hormone imbalances often improves inflammation.

Bone Health

Your body uses calcium to build healthy bones and teeth. Calcium is stored in your bones. A normal part of the aging process is that the bones don't make new bone as fast as they used to when you were younger, so the calcium is taken from the bones instead; you lose bone density this way. And you also lose bone density when you have lower estrogen levels, particularly after menopause. Loss of bone mass over time can lead to osteoporosis, a condition causing the bones to become brittle, weak, and more prone to fracture. A 2015 study reported in the *Journal of Clinical Endocrinology and Metabolism* found that women who have severe hot flashes and night sweats during their transition to menopause usually have more bone loss and are at higher risk for hip fractures than women with less severe symptoms. But the root of all these symptoms may be in the gut.

Low Libido

My husband and I have been married for twenty years, and I loved sex—it was never an issue. And now I would literally rather turn on the nightly news and get depressed about the state of the world than jump into bed. It's like a joke with my friends that we used to sit around and talk about our sex lives, but now all we talk about is how much we're aching and creaking! But since my libido is shot all to hell—and I never thought I'd be saying this—our crummy sex life isn't as big a problem for me as I thought it would be because I just don't care anymore.

—Geri Green, age 58

Your libido is in full force when your sex hormones are balanced. Low testosterone, low progesterone, low estradiol—these hormone deficiencies can put your sex life on hold, much like this patient has said.

Understanding these hormone levels and feeling good about your body go hand in hand (along with a strong relationship)—that is the formula for great sex. But if your hormonal symptoms are interfering with how you feel about yourself, sex and intimacy go out the window. Perimenopause and menopause should be the time of your life when sex is the most FUN—you've got bedroom cred, finally! By this time there is also no fear of pregnancy, plus you really know yourself by now. But when the hormone equilibrium fails you, you may feel more like a nun than a hot Superwoman. And there can be a massive fallout from that, if you know what I mean.

Mood Shifts

I am a monster. I am just full of rage and an angry bitch all the time. My husband said to please fix me or we're going to get divorced, because I'm turning into a different version of me. I'm not nice to him. I'm not nice to anyone. I don't know why. I don't want to be like this anymore, but I just can't help it. I never used to be like this!

—Lisa Fry, age 31

This is a common feeling. Anxiety, anger, crying spells, depression, and irritability can all be signs that your hormones are off. It breaks my heart to see so many patients crying all the time. They are supersensitive to all sorts of triggers—triggers that normally wouldn't send them into a spiral of moodiness and unhappiness, and that saps their ability to handle stress or meet life's challenges.

For Rock Stars and Hustlers, mood shifts can last for a few days; maybe it's a few weeks for Superwomen or Commanders. It all depends on where you are in your menstrual cycle and which hormone is triggering the symptoms. If a typical cycle is twenty-eight days, some women will feel bad when their estrogen spikes on days 1 to 14. For others, the mood shift happens when the progesterone drops on days 14 to 28. Or, one month you might be okay and then the next month it might be a progesterone thing, and then the following month there might be an estrogen thing. This unpredictability can leave you frustrated and wondering if things will ever get better. (Yes, they will!)

These mood shifts are not limited to anxiety and depression; for some women, there can be a full-out flare-up of OCD (obsessive compulsive disorder), bipolar disorder, and ADHD (attention deficit and hyperactivity disorder). As the hormones shift, these mood and neurocognitive symptoms can come and go. For some of my patients, they disappear when the women reach their twenties and then reappear when they are in their fifties. "Why do I feel like a teenager again?" a patient recently asked.

Perimenopause

Perimenopause, which literally means "around menopause," takes place when your female hormones begin to decline—the time between your reproductive years and menopause. You might barely notice it at first, or you might have obvious signs, such as changes to a previously clockwork menstrual cycle, some mood swings, your first hot flash, or any of the other symptoms mentioned in Chapter 1, especially concerning Superstars and Superwomen.

Every woman's perimenopausal period is different. It can start in your mid-thirties or not until your fifties; it can last for a few months or go on for many years. And the symptoms can be anywhere from barely noticeable (if you're one of the lucky ones and follow the advice in this book!) to severely disturbing to your quality of life. For most women, perimenopause lasts an average of four years.

I meet women every day in some phase of their perimenopause who feel like they are going insane. But as we work to identify their key hormone patterns and strive to achieve balance, they get back to their superpowered selves.

PCOS

Polycystic ovary syndrome (PCOS) is one of the most common hormone disorders in women during their reproductive years. While there may be a genetic predisposition to PCOS, the rising rates of this disease imply that there are dietary, lifestyle, and environmental factors also involved.

PCOS appears when inflammation and increased insulin secretion cause changes in ovarian function, affecting ovulation, fertility, weight, and hair. There can be rapid weight gain, acne, hair loss or excessive hair growth on the face, joint pain, and even a decrease in ability to focus and concentrate—these are all symptoms of PCOS. It really is an autoimmune disease. For this reason, many endocrinologists and physicians believe it is named incorrectly—it really is more of a metabolic disorder, rather than a pure hormone disorder.

Clinically, to be diagnosed with PCOS you need to have two of the following: high androgen levels, high insulin levels, ovarian cysts, and/or anovulatory cycles (when an egg is not released by the ovaries during your monthly cycle). PCOS is closely related to endometriosis, with similar hormone patterns and metabolic shifting.

By identifying the hormone patterns and underlying drivers of the inflammation and insulin resistance, we have been able to reverse PCOS and keep it well managed. Happy periods, happy hair, skin, a healthy weight, and a few babies—check!

PMS

Can I get a doctor's excuse for that time of the month? For every month? I am always doubled over in pain. I can't work, I can't focus, I pop Advil all day long and then my stomach hurts. I don't want to be seen like this.

—Dara Lee, age 29

The cramps, the chocolate and salt cravings, the wanting to hide—who has not suffered from premenstrual syndrome (PMS)?

Post-ovulation, or in the middle of your cycle, estrogen and progesterone levels start to drop, triggering your menstrual flow. But when the balance of estrogen and progesterone is off, or there is a high load of inflammation in the body, you may experience cramps, heavy bleeding, and pain that can keep you hiding at home.

The most common physical PMS symptoms are swollen or tender breasts, constipation or diarrhea, bloating, cramps (which can be completely debilitating), headache or backache, exhaustion or lack of energy, clumsiness, and a lower tolerance for noise or light. There are other emotional and physical symptoms as well, including irritability, anger, sleep problems (sleeping too much or too little), appetite changes and food cravings (please pass the chips) caused by a shift in electrolytes and blood sugar as a result of the hormone imbalance. And the list continues: trouble with concentration or memory, mood swings, tension or anxiety, depression, feelings of sadness, crying spells, and lack of sexual desire. You are no longer you—for however long this PMS lasts.

Fortunately, when you balance your estrogen and progesterone levels, the intensity of these PMS symptoms reduces and can even go away. When this happens, that time of the month becomes just another day on the calendar.

Skin Changes

I have important events to go to for work, but I can't find an outfit that covers my psoriasis. I have white flaky patches all over my arms, legs, and even my scalp. This started three months after I went into menopause, and none of the medications I've been prescribed have helped at all.

—Jada Love, age 51

The loss of estrogen and progesterone impacts skin health. Collagen production slows down and fat loss increases, changing the structure of the face and the firmness of the skin. Wrinkling, easy bruising, and drooping jowls are all part of the hormone decline that comes with age.

Many women run for cosmetic dermatology procedures, use skincare products and devices, have surgeries, or do anything else to restore what they once had. But restoring your hormone balance, achieving a healthy gut function, and optimizing your nutrient levels will treat these beauty concerns from the inside out.

Sleep Issues

I've never been able to nap. Not even when I was in kindergarten and our teacher told us to rest and snooze! So when I was in my mid-forties, I started having a real problem because I would wake up every single night at 3:48 a.m. and be up till, literally, 5:14. Down to the minute, believe it or not. It didn't matter what time I'd go to bed or how tired I was; I'd still wake up. I was just exhausted and cranky all the time, but I still couldn't nap. Finally, one of my exasperated friends told me to go on HRT and see if that would help. It worked! It only took about a week before I was sleeping soundly again.

—Lily Shag, age 57

As you know by now, your sleep cycle is regulated by cortisol, which should spike early in the morning to get you out of bed, and melatonin, which should spike in the evening to allow you to wind down. But as your estrogen and progesterone levels decline with age, cortisol spikes to wake you up—you guessed it—between 2 and 4 a.m. That's what jolted my patient awake at 3:48 a.m.

Sleep complaints are so common in the women who come to my practice. Not only is their cortisol spiking when it shouldn't be, but they've also often been self-medicating with sleeping pills—when what they really need is hormone balancing instead. These sleeping pills can range from Benadryl, an antihistamine that makes you sleepy, to over-the-counter melatonin in high doses, to prescription medications that can quickly become addictive and disrupt your natural sleep cycle. Tapering off these pills can take anywhere from a couple of weeks to a full *year*. It's incredibly frustrating for women to be given a prescription for sleeping pills that takes months and months to get out of their system, when simple hormone balancing may be the long-term answer.

Thyroid Disorders

Thyroid disorders are not unusual, and they are vastly underdiagnosed in women. It's estimated that around 20 million Americans have some form of a thyroid disease, with up to 60 percent of those unaware that they even have the condition. Women are five to eight times more likely than men to develop these thyroid conditions because we are more susceptible to autoimmune diseases and inflammation—the root cause of many thyroid conditions. We are also often dealing with an enormous amount of stress, which taxes the adrenal glands. Increased levels of cortisol force the thyroid to work harder and eventually trigger hypothyroidism. In addition, stress depletes important nutrients from the body that would keep the thyroid and the adrenals in balance.

There are several types of thyroid disorder:

> *Hyperthyroidism*, or an overactive thyroid, can be caused by nodules on the thyroid, inflammation, or excessive iodine intake, along with a genetic predisposition. Most often it is caused by Graves' disease, an autoimmune disorder triggering hormone overproduction. Environmental toxins, including heavy metals and endocrine disrupters, may also be responsible for an overactive thyroid.

> *Hypothyroidism*, or an underactive thyroid, occurs when you don't have enough of the thyroid hormones. This can be the result of genetics, pregnancy, extreme stress, or medications. Of the 60 percent of those who don't know they have thyroid issues, hypothyroidism is the main culprit.

> *Hashimoto's disease* is a genetic autoimmune disease that occurs when your thyroid becomes inflamed and your

immune system mistakenly attacks it. It's the primary cause of hypothyroidism in the United States. As it progresses, it is often characterized by a swelling at the front of the throat, and it typically progresses slowly over time, leading to a drop in thyroid hormone levels in your body.

- *Goiters/nodules and thyroid cysts.* Inflammation in the thyroid gland can present in a number of ways other than an alteration in thyroid function. I meet many patients who have normal thyroid function but have enlarged thyroids or goiters, or cysts or nodules that have to be watched. Conventionally, these may get dismissed until they are past a certain size, but for the EastWest approach, inflammation, nutrient deficiencies, and genetics are at work, warning us to stay on top of our thyroid health.

Vaginal Changes

I cannot get another UTI. I'm on my fourth round of antibiotics in six months—because I get a urinary tract infection every time I have sex. Not to mention that sex really hurts.

—*Mary Singh, age 26*

What can be one of the most painful symptoms of hormonal decline and shifting lies within your vagina. As your estrogen levels go down, so does the natural lubrication and the thickness of the vaginal walls. Dryness can make sex very uncomfortable. Fortunately, regular use of lubricants can help, as can prescription vaginal estrogen creams that can be inserted up to twice a week to build the tissues back up and provide more lubrication.

Another hormonal symptom can be a changing pH, leading to a shift in your vaginal microbiome. That occurs when urinary tract infections can be more prevalent owing to thinner vaginal walls that make it easier for unwanted bugs to proliferate. Always see your gynecologist if you have any persistent symptoms like pain, itching, redness, or discharge.

Weight Gain

Why do I have a beer belly when I don't even drink beer? Why am I gaining weight when I haven't changed anything—I eat the same and work out the same but I can't lose an ounce, let alone a pound.

—Maya Sims, age 41

I hear comments like this practically every day. As women enter perimenopause, they can experience anywhere from a five- to eight-pound weight gain, with much of it around the belly. For some women, the numbers are even higher—close to fifteen to twenty pounds. I also see friends and colleagues whose weight remained stable for decades, but then they become completely bewildered at how their bodies are changing. A belly suddenly appears and won't go away.

While it's important to remember that you can be healthy at many different weights and in many different dress sizes, a change in your standard or stable weight is alarming to most women, so they try to overcorrect with extreme diets and workouts, which don't work.

There are two reasons for this weight gain:

Hormone loss, especially of estrogen and progesterone, creates a natural tendency for us to become insulin resistant, which means the body isn't processing insulin efficiently, leading to more circulating blood sugar, which is then stored as fat (most often belly fat).

- With the loss of hormones there also comes a loss of muscle mass. This leads to a decline in resting metabolic rate, meaning the body needs fewer calories every day—even if you think it doesn't. Women and men also become less active as they enter their forties and fifties; even if you weren't running marathons, you were probably running after children or were just more active in general. There is also more stress from taking care of children, family, and busy careers.

Why Is This Weight Gain in Your Belly?

Abdominal fat or visceral fat (the fat around our organs) develops as we become more insulin resistant, meaning that our average blood sugars are higher than before. There are also shifts in the microbiome (gut bacteria) that trigger fat storage in the abdomen and other end organs.

What does this mean for women with hormone shifts? The first response is to usually starve or skip meals. But this short-term fix ultimately leads to weight gain, since doing this slows your metabolic rate. Over-exercising drives your cortisol levels up and triggers inflammation, and then it worsens insulin resistance. So what to do? You do structured eating, as I lay out in my Thirty-Day Hormone Reset (Chapter 9) to uncover your sweet spot and keep all that visceral fat at bay.

For me, at least, the notion of an unavoidable middle-age spread is total myth. The weight gain is connected to hormones and to gut function—and to muscle mass. The complex relationships among hormone levels, metabolism, gut health, and stress or other lifestyle factors is mind-boggling. Yet putting the pieces of this puzzle together is exactly what we do when using the Thirty-Day Hormone Reset (Chapter 9).

Do These Symptoms Sound Familiar? Which Ones Are You Struggling with the Most?

Women may have many of these symptoms, or have a few over time, or even—if you're lucky and take excellent care of yourself—none at all. In my experience working with women of all ages, I've found that lower energy levels, sleep disruption, and irregular periods are the three most common symptoms of hormone shifting. Everything else (like anxiety, depression, and fatigue) starts to follow in a domino effect. There is a correlation between having a symptom-laden perimenopausal transition and having a problematic menopausal transition—but only if you do nothing about it.

Furthermore, these are not the only hormone-based conditions we see in our practice; I did not discuss autoimmune diseases and hormone-based cancers, nor everything from lupus, rheumatoid arthritis, Crohn's disease, and ulcerative colitis, all of which have hormone triggers, or at least a hormone puzzle piece. Breast cancer, thyroid cancer, endometrial cancer—those are really easy to link to changing hormones levels. But all these conditions could veer in a different direction if we thought more critically about hormones and how they interface with other elements of the body.

EastWest medicine does exactly this. It provides answers as we all try to tip the scales toward optimal health. I mentioned that this book was about the Journey UP. And it is—up and away from a list of conditions and disorders and toward a balanced, healthy life.

So, take another look at your Hormone Symptom Checklist (page 62). No matter how many symptoms you've marked, you can take steps to start feeling more like yourself again. It's not you—*it's your hormones*.

Now that you have a clear picture of your symptoms and you understand that they're connected to your hormones, it's time to dig deeper. A foundational knowledge of the hormones themselves is essential to learning how to balance your body. You will understand what they do behind the scenes and how their imbalances can have a domino effect. In fact, you can think of "hormones" as a language your body is using to communicate with you. Now you are going to learn how to speak that language.

Let's get on to the nitty-gritty details about your hormones. Ready to geek out? Welcome to Hormone University.

chapter 3

Hormone University

Hormones, Hormone Testing, and HRT

To understand hormone shifts, you have to understand hormones: who and what they are, how they work, and how they make you feel. Welcome to Hormone University, where I lay out the essentials—everything you need to know about your hormones.

What Is a Hormone?

That seems like a ridiculous question, but it's an important one. Hormones are your body's chemical messengers sent out to various organs to dictate various functions. Hormones are made and manufactured in the gut and liver, with the influence of certain other organs depending on the hormone. The hormones are then released into the bloodstream to do their jobs. There are over fifty different hormones identified in the human body, and likely more that have yet to be identified. There are also multiple networks, organs, and systems involved in the management of these hormones.

Your body needs certain nutrients, such as vitamins and minerals, to manufacture those hormones and to metabolize them properly. Fat is also high on the list of required nutrients, as it is crucial for this process to work properly. That is why women who are severely underweight stop getting their periods—they don't have enough estrogen—while women who are severely overweight often have too much estrogen, as it is stored in body fat. So, when you think about nutrition, it's not just about how much you weigh but also about the essential nutrients you must ingest for a smoothly running metabolism.

All hormone production naturally decreases as we age, no matter how well we eat or take care of ourselves. That's even more reason to do as much as you can, no matter what age, to regulate your hormones as much as you can.

Different areas of the body are responsible for producing or processing different hormones. Let's take a look:

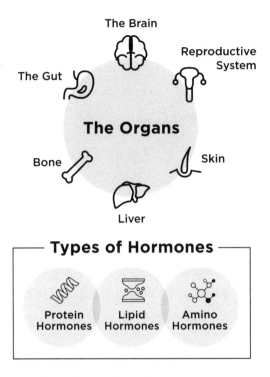

The Organs

The Brain

Reproductive System

The Gut

Bone

Skin

Liver

Types of Hormones

Protein Hormones

Lipid Hormones

Amino Hormones

The 7 Major Hormones

- Estrogen
- DHEA
- Progesterone
- Testosterone
- Cortisol
- Thyroid Hormones
- Insulin

In the next section, I describe all the major hormones so you can better understand what each is actually doing in the body. These are the hormones you need to know, and you'll learn how to balance them in the Thirty-Day Hormone Reset (Chapter 9).

Note: To see the specific hormone tests and levels I recommend for each shift, see the section "The Hormone Tests You Need" (page 121), later in this chapter.

Stress and Sleep Hormones

Cortisol

Cortisol is known as the stress hormone. Like all hormones, it needs to be in just the right amount to work well. Too much cortisol and you feel the stress, such as in heart palpitations, anxiety, or trouble sleeping. Too little cortisol and you are chronically tired or crave salt, and then the body starts to break down. First comes the leaky gut, next inflammation, and then the intensity of your symptoms picks up.

Where It's Made

In your adrenal glands, located above your kidneys.

How It's Measured

Morning cortisol levels can be measured with a blood test, but at other times the cortisol levels are variable, so conventional lab testing is often not helpful. I check saliva levels throughout the day to establish a pattern for cortisol regulation. This way, we can determine the cortisol pattern in a twenty-four hour or a three-day sample, which is more important information than presented by a single cortisol level.

What It Does

Cortisol increases the amount of sugars in your body. The right amount of cortisol helps you get moving. Cortisol levels are meant to peak in the morning so you can get up, get out of bed, and do your thing. They gradually decline as the day progresses, winding down as you approach bedtime, and then are replenished as you sleep so you have the higher level again when you wake up.

What Happens When You Don't Have Enough

With too little cortisol, you end up tired all the time, maybe even depressed. You don't have the adrenaline to get up and get moving, leaving you droopy, fatigued, and wanting to isolate from your responsibilities.

What Happens When You Have Too Much

Having too much cortisol for a long of a period of time is defined as *stress*. This can look like anxiety; trouble sleeping, focusing, or concentrating; heart racing; or sweaty palms. Normally, a stressor would spike the cortisol levels later in the day, as with any sort of stimulus, and then the levels go back down. But over a period of time, if the external life stress is too great or lasts for too long, or if the stress is internal, you're lacking certain nutrients, or there's too much inflammation, for example, the cortisol levels remain elevated.

This leaves you with the classic feeling of being wired and tired. You want to go to sleep at night, but you can't because your cortisol levels are high. Or, you fall asleep and wake up between 2 and 4 o'clock in the morning. If this pattern of stress continues and the cortisol levels remain chronically high, every other organ has to compensate. Your body seeks energy from nutrients, gut health, the thyroid, and additional hormones—ultimately leading to full-out depletion of everything and an adrenal crash.

I tell my patients that this develops in stages. Stage one is mild adrenal fatigue whereby you might have an afternoon slump. Stage two is the wired and tired feeling whereby you're up at night and tired all day long. Stage three is when you totally crash out; you're tired all the time because your cortisol levels have plummeted and remain constantly low. You have no energy. Oftentimes, women with this condition even get labeled with depression and are given medication for depression, which does not solve the problem of adrenal fatigue.

Signs of Adrenal Fatigue

There are four key stages of adrenal fatigue:

Stage 1: Tired in the afternoon, 3–5 p.m. crash

Stage 2: Tired all day

Stage 3: Tired all day but up at night

Stage 4: Full-out wired and tired

Symptoms of Adrenal Fatigue

Anxiety and/or repetitive thoughts

IBS—constipation, diarrhea

Insomnia

Low blood pressure

Low blood sugar episodes

Salt cravings

Thinning hair

Adrenaline

Adrenaline is the "fight or flight" hormone.

Where It's Made

Primarily in the adrenal glands.

What It Does

Adrenaline is released to aid your reflexes so you can react quickly when you're in a stressful situation. It increases your heart rate, raises your blood pressure, and boosts your overall energy.

How It's Measured

Adrenaline is measured by looking at catecholamines (the family adrenaline belongs to) in the blood or urine.

What Happens When You Don't Have Enough

Having a low adrenaline level is called adrenal insufficiency, and it usually happens only in rare cases. But when the adrenaline is low, it becomes difficult for the body to produce cortisol, the stress hormone, which leads to low blood pressure, low blood sugar, and more complications.

What Happens When You Have Too Much

As with cortisol, adrenaline levels rise when you have anxiety, although adrenaline peaks last for a shorter time in the body than do cortisol peaks. If adrenaline remains elevated for too long, there are many different symptoms, including an elevated heart rate, high insulin level, high glucose, decreased appetite, and trouble sleeping. You can feel jittery and terrible, and your breathing can get ragged and rapid.

Melatonin

Melatonin is the hormone that regulates your sleep cycle, or the circadian rhythm.

Where It's Made

The pineal gland, located in the center of your brain.

What It Does

Melatonin is usually secreted at night and helps you to fall asleep. It is released in response to light, and so should peak in the evening as the skies darken; it's the flip side of cortisol, which should be highest in the morning.

How It's Measured

Melatonin can be measured in the blood or saliva. As with cortisol, multiple samples are taken throughout the day, with results that are more helpful than a single static level.

What Happens When You Don't Have Enough

Too little melatonin presents sleep challenges, from trouble falling asleep to poor sleep quality. Melatonin is essential for a proper circadian rhythm; for this reason, taking a supplement can be helpful for shift workers, for people suffering jetlag, or for those with difficulty falling asleep, rather than staying asleep.

What Happens When You Have Too Much

Too much melatonin is usually the result of oversupplementation. The side effects of too much melatonin include daytime sleepiness, dizziness, and fatigue.

If you stay up past the point where you're exhausted and know you should go to sleep, your melatonin levels will be disrupted. This makes it harder to then get to sleep. Over time, your natural circadian rhythm will be disrupted, impacting not just your sleep but also the secretion of all your other hormones, as well as your digestive health.

> ### How to Take Melatonin if Necessary
>
> Melatonin is available over the counter in the form of pills and gummies. Don't think, however, that because it is so readily available, you don't need to determine the correct amount for your own sleep needs. I have the same thing to say about melatonin as I say about every other hormone: there's a sweet spot for it. When you take too much of any hormone, the supplement takes over your body's natural ability to produce it, and this messes with the signaling. That's why some experts advise against taking melatonin every day or to take it only under a doctor's supervision. I believe that low doses (1 to 3 milligrams daily) will give you a slow release that won't shut down your own production of melatonin. Taking more than that will not be helpful.

Metabolism Hormones

Insulin

This is the hormone that regulates your blood sugar, pushing glucose into the cells.

Where It's Made

In the beta cells of the pancreas.

What It Does

Insulin is responsible for fat storage and is a large player in overall metabolic health. In an ideal situation, you eat, insulin is released in response to your circulating blood sugar, or glucose level—which is the fuel for your body—and then this glucose is delivered into the appropriate cells where energy is needed, and the result is satisfaction. The balances among circulating blood sugar, insulin secretion from the pancreas, hunger, and appetite are all in tune when the body is healthy, without stress or hormone disruption. (I know, a.k.a. never!)

In addition to the pancreas, other organs regulate the insulin, including the liver, muscles, and your digestive system. All these organs are assisting and helping in the management of blood glucose, thereby signaling insulin release and function.

Step #2
PANCREAS
The pancreas (the body's glucose monitor) detects the glucose.

Step #1
CONSUME
The food we consume becomes glucose and enters the bloodstream.

Once energy is depleted, it's time to eat and begin the cycle again!

How
Insulin
Works

Step #3
INSULIN
The pancreas releases the hormone insulin, unlocking the body's cells to let in glucose.

Step #4
CELLS
Once glucose is in the cells, the cells turn it into energy.

Step #5
ENERGY
Energy fuels the body and blood sugar decreases until we eat again to refuel.

How It's Measured

The best tests for insulin are fasting blood glucose and a hemoglobin A1C. Serum or blood levels of insulin and C-peptide are helpful, as well.

What Happens When You Don't Have Enough

Low insulin levels keep too much glucose in your bloodstream and send not enough to your cells, which means you end up with hyperglycemia. Symptoms of hyperglycemia include sweating, dizziness or feeling shaky, and/or agitation or nervousness. Having low insulin is often an issue for Type 1 diabetics.

What Happens When You Have Too Much

High insulin levels occur from eating too much or eating foods that are toxic or taxing on the body. This leads to a disproportionately exaggerated response of insulin. You've doubtless experienced this when you eat a meal that is primarily simple carbohydrates—a bagel with cream cheese and jelly, for example—which is quickly converted into glucose. An hour or so later, you're hungry again. In addition, from a blood sugar standpoint, refined foods, processed foods, and foods with a lot of dyes, chemicals, and additives raise the blood sugar levels even higher than do whole foods.

Having an exaggerated insulin response occasionally is no big deal for most people. But when it happens multiple times throughout the day, for years and years, you can develop insulin resistance. This resistance happens when the insulin levels stay elevated and continue to push glucose into the cells. But since this is too much fuel to be used up at that time, something has to happen to that excess glucose; you guessed it—it's stored as fat.

Insulin release isn't just about what happens in your pancreas, however. There's a relationship between the secretion of insulin from the pancreas and levels of blood glucose that the liver, kidneys, and gut influence as well. For instance, the liver regulates glucose by producing the hormone glucagon, which the liver releases when it senses hypoglycemia. But if you have a "dirty" liver that isn't processing hormones properly (which you'll read about in Chapter 8), you'll have an impaired glucose response, with levels that might be too high or are made at the wrong time.

As mentioned, the gut is responsible for insulin regulation as well. Gut bacteria, or the microbiome as we like to call it, regulate blood glucose levels by sensing nutrient levels in the gut and blood sugar levels in the liver. Also, the kidneys release blood glucose depending on what the body is doing or take up glucose and reabsorb it, destroying the insulin.

The relationships among the gut, liver, pancreas, and hormones are recognized in the EastWest approach, which considers these factors in hormone management.

Thyroid Hormones (T3, T4, TSH, TRH)

Of all the body's hormones, those produced by the thyroid gland are the most talked about and the most misunderstood, especially for women. Didn't I mention medical gaslighting earlier? I don't know how many missed cases of hypothyroidism, Hashimoto's disease, Graves' disease, and goiters I have seen in my clinics. When you're being told that your thyroid levels are normal, but you still have many different and often debilitating symptoms, you absolutely need to ask for more advanced testing from a medical practitioner who will listen to you. Especially if the symptoms listed here are ones you may be experiencing.

I discuss this in more detail in the coming chapter on hormone symptoms and conditions, as there's just not enough conversation about how the thyroid actually works, all the different types of thyroid disorders, whether they are genetic or not, or how stress plays into them, as well as how critical the nutrient load is and the importance of gut health. I could go on and on, but we will get there—I promise!

Where It's Made

T3, T4, and TSH

Signals from the hypothalamus and the pituitary glands are sent to the small, butterfly-shaped thyroid gland located at the base of the front of the neck to produce the key thyroid hormones: T3, T4, and TSH. Some of this manufacturing also takes place in the gut, as the microbiome determines the conversion of T4—the less active thyroid hormone—into T3. There is also recent research on the role of T1 and T2—thyroid hormones that are being explored in terms of their function and relevance.

TRH

This is the hormone produced by the hypothalamus that signals the release of TSH from the pituitary and then the release of thyroid hormones from the thyroid.

What They Do

These hormones regulate your metabolism, including how well you burn calories. Thyroid hormones impact and influence so many different aspects of your health—your energy, mood, memory, gut health, hair and skin, eyebrows and eyelashes.

The thyroid's hormones, like all other hormones in the body, work in concert with insulin, cortisol, estrogen, and progesterone. Indeed, we find this over and over again in practice. For example, your thyroid efficiency is directly related to your adrenals and to the release of cortisol and adrenaline. When your adrenals and other organs are stressed or taxed, this can trigger a thyroid dysfunction. Also, if your estrogen levels get too high, the thyroid has to work even harder to produce its hormones.

How They Are Measured

Blood tests measure the levels of T3, T4, and TSH in your body. In practice, we also measure RT3, along with total and free levels of T3 and T4. RT3 is known as a reverse thyroid hormone and will bind to iodine receptors. It is typically high when the body is under stress or undergoing a prolonged illness. Total T3 and T4 refers to the amount of this hormone that is both freely floating and the amount bound to the proteins. Both are needed for optimal thyroid hormone function.

But here is where you may need to advocate for yourself. Because your thyroid function is unique to you, it is way too easy to accept good news when told you're fine even though you're not. We are learning more and more that people have their own "normal." Conventionally, blood work is ordered for the T3, T4, and TSH levels only, but these tests don't look at all the different metabolites of the thyroid hormones or the thyroid antibodies, and so they cannot pinpoint what type of thyroid condition or disease you might be dealing with.

For example, the normal range for TSH is 0.5 to 5.0 mIU/L (milli–international units per liter). Let's say your TSH is 3.5. You've been told it's normal, but that 3.5 is still not optimal for you—you may be hypothyroid or have low thyroid function even at this "normal" number. And if your thyroid antibody load is high—antithyroglobulin ab and thyroid peroxidase antibodies—that means you're still dealing with chronic inflammation and need to be more aggressive with your treatment. But from what I see in my day-to-day interactions with patients, this testing is often missed, and patients and doctors are led to believe they are "fine."

In addition, many women are prescribed thyroid medication for years, but they actually have Hashimoto's disease, which is an inflammatory condition. Thus, they need more support than just thyroid medication.

What Happens When You Don't Have Enough

An underactive thyroid, or hypothyroidism, occurs when you don't have enough of the thyroid hormones you need. You can have a wide range of symptoms, such as weight gain, fatigue, fertility issues, feeling cold all the time, and more.

What Happens When You Have Too Much

An overactive thyroid, or hyperthyroidism, triggers overproduction of thyroid hormones. This can cause weight loss, irritability, vision loss, fatigue, sleep issues, and mood swings.

Sex Hormones

Estrogen

Estrogen is the primary and ultimate female hormone.

Where It's Made

Primarily in your ovaries, but estrogen is also secreted from your uterus and from body fat. It gets directed by FSH (follicle stimulating hormone) that is secreted by the pituitary gland, which in turn gets its directions from GnRH (gonadotropin-releasing hormone), which is secreted by the hypothalamus.

What It Does

Estrogen helps trigger puberty, prepares the uterus and body for pregnancy, and regulates the menstrual cycle. Levels of estrogen build during the first two weeks of your cycle and then lower during the second half (days 14 to 28). You need the right amount of estrogen to build up your endometrial lining, have a monthly period, and be fertile; you also need enough estrogen to have good skin, hair, brain function, cognition, and bone health.

How It's Measured

There are three types of estrogen: estradiol, estrone, and estriol. These can all be measured in the blood or saliva. There is a lot of discussion about when to measure these, since their levels do fluctuate; many recommend testing on days 19 to 21 (the luteal phase). In our practice, we have established that estradiol levels should not be below 50 nor above 200. Estrone, the storage form of estrogen, should not be above 150.

What Happens When You Don't Have Enough

Without normal levels of estrogen, your menstrual cycle will be irregular or cease altogether. You can also experience dry skin, dry hair, and more fatigue or depression. As the amount of estrogen continues to lower, there is a greater risk for osteoporosis, dementia, altered gut health, and cardiometabolic profiles.

What Happens When You Have Too Much

Too much estrogen, or estrogen dominance, leads to a thickened uterine lining that can trigger spotting, heavy periods, fibroids, and ovarian cysts, as well as migraines, other headaches, anxiety, depression, brain fog, and joint pain. Tender breasts, bloating, and constipation are also signs of estrogen dominance.

Progesterone

Progesterone is a critical anti-inflammatory hormone that does not get enough press. Its levels increase in the second half of the menstrual cycle, and as it falls, it triggers the menstrual flow. Additional progesterone hormones include pregnenalone and 17-hydroxprogesterone.

Where It's Made

Progesterone is made in the ovaries after signaling from the pituitary hormone lutropin, or leutinizing hormone (LH), which also gets direction from GnRH, the hypothalamic hormone.

What It Does

Progesterone is needed for your menstrual cycle and to sustain a pregnancy. It triggers the second half of your monthly menstrual cycle, helps to balance estrogen levels, and regulates mood, sleep, energy, and even fluid levels in the body. It is also anti-inflammatory and helps to manage the gut microbiome, which many women aren't aware of. The ultimate calming hormone, progesterone is critical in helping you manage stress, but at the same time it gets depleted when you are stressed for far too long. I know this one well; I crashed my progesterone levels in my twenties and needed progesterone replacement to get back on track.

How It's Measured

Progesterone levels can be measured in blood and saliva, with saliva more helpful as it can be collected multiple measures during the day, rather than reflecting one static level, which can be misleading. In my practice, I established blood levels of progesterone to be above 0.5 but not greater than 25.

What Happens When You Don't Have Enough

When levels of progesterone drop, there is more chance of anxiety, shortened menstrual cycles, and sleep disturbances (hello, 3 a.m.!). And this begins a vicious cycle of stress, causing progesterone levels to be rapidly depleted, which then triggers more stress and anxiety, since progesterone is the anti-inflammatory and calming hormone.

What Happens When You Have Too Much

Too much progesterone gives you that heavy, pregnant feeling. Many women feel like they are walking through mud, or are foggy, feel heavy, or gaining weight rapidly. Metabolizing and balancing your progesterone levels is just as important as metabolizing and balancing your estrogen levels.

Androgens

Just as men have low levels of female hormones, women have low levels of androgens, or the typically male hormones. These hormones include testosterone, DHEA (dehydroepiandrosterone), DHT (dihydrotestosterone), 17-hydroxyprogesterone, and androstenedione.

Where It's Made

Primarily in the ovaries, with smaller amounts secreted from the adrenal glands and fat cells.

What It Does

Androgens play a role in gender characteristics, overall hormone balance, and hormone breakdown. They kick-start puberty and are responsible for facial, underarm, and pubic hair. Further, they are involved in the health of the muscles, liver, and bones.

How They Are Measured

Androgens are typically measured in the blood or saliva, with blood giving more static values and saliva giving values in a pattern over time.

What Happens When You Don't Have Enough

Low androgen levels can cause low libido, bone loss, and hot flashes. Androgen deficiency can also delay puberty and dampen libido.

What Happens When You Have Too Much

Androgen levels seem to be increasing in women. From early puberty to acne and issues with ovulation and infertility, we are seeing an explosion of problems caused by androgen excess. As women age, falling levels of estrogen and progesterone can allow androgen dominance, resulting in late-onset acne and male-pattern balding. Excess androgens can also trigger insulin resistance or high blood sugars, impacting all hormones. Androgen levels increase with stress, poor sleep, nutrient-depleted diets, processed foods, and trauma. There's even a neuro-inflammatory component, with androgen-related anxiety, depression, and trouble focusing. Androgens and androgen sensitivity are responsible for the rise in PCOS, hair loss, thyroid conditions, and infertility.

Brain Hormones—Hypothalamic and Pituitary

You may not realize how essential your brain is to hormone regulation. The hypothalamus and pituitary glands sit close by one another in the brain and are influenced by stress, sleep, trauma, medications, and so much more. Hormones produced by these glands direct the other hormones discussed here about how to do their job. But, if your brain is anything like mine, those directions don't always get followed and the command center—well, it's not always turned on.

Hypothalamic Pituitary Axis

Follicle-Stimulating Hormone and Luteinizing Hormone

Where They Are Made

Both hormones are made in the pituitary gland.

What They Do

During your menstrual cycle, the follicle-stimulating hormone (FSH) stimulates the ovarian follicle, causing an egg to grow and more estrogen to be produced. This then triggers the pituitary to stop making the FSH and start making more luteinizing hormone (LH). When this happens, you ovulate; your egg is released and your progesterone levels go up. If you don't become pregnant, the progesterone levels drop, you get your period, and the cycle starts all over again.

How They Are Measured

These hormones are measured with a blood test or a urine test. If you're testing for fertility reasons, you may need to give samples over a certain period of time.

What Happens When You Don't Have Enough

You may be having fertility issues and find it hard to become pregnant. Low FSH levels often correlate with pituitary failure and failure to ovulate. Low FSH levels are common in PCOS as well, when ovulation is often disrupted.

What Happens When You Have Too Much

Having too much FSH is rare, but for those who do have that situation, it's often a sign of menopause or low ovarian reserves and poor egg quality. It implies that your body is needing more FSH to stimulate ovulation. High LH levels are often found in PCOS, blocking ovulation.

Your Menstrual Cycle

There are two phases to the menstrual cycle: (1) when the egg is about to be released and estrogen levels rise; and (2) after the release, when progesterone levels rise in preparation for potential fertilization. The average cycle is twenty-eight to thirty-four days, but this time can vary a lot.

- Day 1 of your cycle is the first day you have a flow of blood. Even if your cycle is erratic, you still start counting from the first day of bleeding. Just so you know, spotting and bleeding aren't the same. Spotting is just droplets here and there; menstrual bleeding is true, continuous flow. And when there is flow, a few new eggs begin to grow in your ovaries and the uterine lining thickens. This is the follicular phase, during which time estrogen levels are rising.
- About two to three weeks later, one (or more) mature egg is released from the ovary during ovulation and passes into the fallopian tubes. This is the luteal phase, with higher progesterone levels that enable fertilization, if there are any sperm swimming around.
- If there's no fertilization, the egg dies and the estrogen and progesterone levels drop. The thick lining of the uterus is shed in your next menstrual flow. Then the cycle starts all over again.

Growth Hormone

Where It's Made

The growth hormone (GH) is secreted by the pituitary gland.

What It Does

As the name implies, GH is responsible for growth in children, but it also regulates metabolism in adults. Muscle mass, fluid balance, and bone health are all affected by the growth hormones.

How It's Measured

GH can be measured using IGF1 (insulin-like growth factor 1) levels in the blood.

GnRH

Where It's Made

Gonadotropin-releasing hormone (GnRH) is produced by the hypothalamus.

What It Does

GnRH directs production of the pituitary hormones FSH and LH so they can do their jobs. It can be measured in the blood, but is a little more difficult to check.

ACTH

Where It's Made

The adrenocorticotropic hormone (ACTH) is secreted by the pituitary gland.

What It Does

ACTH signals the cortisol and adrenaline production from the adrenal glands. Given this function, ACTH plays a role in stress management and is a part of the hypothalamic-pituitary-adrenal axis that ultimately affects all hormone levels.

How It's Measured

ACTH can be measured in blood tests.

Prolactin

Where It's Made

Prolactin (PRL) is released by the pituitary gland.

What It Does

Prolactin stimulates breast development and milk production in women. When it is in excess levels, it also functions as an androgen—and often it is elevated in PCOS.

How It's Measured

Prolactin can be measured in blood tests.

What Is Hormone Replacement Therapy?

When your estrogen and progesterone levels aren't normal, hormone replacement therapy (HRT) can be prescribed to ease some or all of the symptoms, especially if the symptoms are severe or are interfering with your quality of life. However, HRT should not be a considered a quick fix. When you know the basics of the EastWest approach to hormone balancing (discussed in several chapters that follow), you'll have a deeper understanding of how the hormones being prescribed will affect the rest of your body, particularly your liver and gut. But I explain more about the EastWest approach in Chapter 5.

During perimenopause and menopause, your doctor may suggest HRT when your levels of estrogen and progesterone are fluctuating or decreasing. You will have your levels tested and then decide with your medical practitioner what form of therapy might be best for you. HRT is available in pill form, as skin patches, gels, rings, and vaginal creams. Most HRT contains both estrogen and progesterone, but formulations can differ based on your needs.

About Hormone Replacement Therapy

One of the biggest setbacks in hormonal treatment came about thanks to a distinctly flawed study of hormone replacement therapy (HRT) that caused screaming headlines and panic around the world, and it continues to cause women to fear hormones.

Initiated by a division of the National Institutes of Health, the Women's Health Initiative Study monitored 27,347 U.S. women ages fifty to seventy-nine who had enrolled in hormone trials between the years 1993 and 1998. The focus was on investigating whether the effects of combined hormones or estrogen alone could prevent coronary heart disease and osteoporosis, and if there was an associated risk for breast cancer. Women in the study took hormone pills or a placebo, and they were expecting to be tracked for many years.

Researchers soon found that instead of there being a decreased risk, the rates of overall illnesses and death, particularly of estrogen-based diseases like breast cancer, were 12 percent higher in women taking the estrogen plus progestin than in women taking the placebo. When the news came out that the estrogen-plus-progestin and estrogen-alone trials had been stopped early (in July 2002 and March 2004, respectively), doctors were stunned and women were terrified. They had been told that HRT was good for their health and strengthened their bones. Instead, this study implied that HRT was a risk factor for early death.

What was the biggest flaw in this study? It tracked *postmenopausal women* only! These women already had low levels of estrogen and progesterone. The estrogen these women were given was Premarin, synthesized from horse urine, which isn't even an estrogen that biochemically and structurally resembles what women naturally make in their bodies.

Over twenty years later, many women are still afraid of doing HRT in any form, owing to the hysteria that arose about this study. Lost in the media firestorm were the findings that women in their fifties who took estrogen alone had a 16 percent *reduced* risk of overall illness and death. In fact, it was the women in their seventies who took estrogen alone who had a 17 percent increased risk of overall illness.

Since then, researchers have found that women really need hormones. Brain volume decreases without hormones. Vibrant hair and skin, libido, cognitive function, joint health, bone health, and energy levels—are all highly dependent on hormonal health.

So, hormones and HRT should not be feared. Over two decades ago, I had to go on bio-identical progesterone (BHT). The cumulative effects of stress and poor diet, altered sleep patterns, and poor gut health had left my body depleted. I did not, like many of the women I continue to meet, have the raw materials to make hormones on my own. I took progesterone for about six months. But as I learned to rebalance my body, replenish my nutrients, restore my gut health and sleep, and balance my other hormones, I found I didn't need it anymore. My journey made it clear: I need to be gluten-free, balance my thyroid hormones, supplement my diet with protein and B vitamins, and get good sleep to have happy hormones. When the synergy of biochemistry works, hormones and hormone replacement therapy add to our superpowers.

As with all medications, there can be risks with HRT, as I mentioned in Chapter 1. When HRT is prescribed with a one-size-fits-all, aggressive approach, that should signal caution. The increased risk of blood clots, breast cancer, gallbladder disease, heart attack, or stroke is small, but it is still something to be considered. This is why I prefer bio-identical hormones, whereby I can tweak the doses and start with very low doses that do, indeed, give the desired clinical benefits and improved quality of life.

These bio-identical formulations usually have more protective estrogen (estriol) than estradiol, which is more biologically active but also has to be watched more carefully. If the bio-identicals aren't working and I'm not seeing results, though, I'll go to some of the conventional hormone formulations, like prescription estrogen patches, which are gentler than pills using Premarin. This approach usually works beautifully as long as I am constantly monitoring my estrogen levels.

There are pros and cons to HRT, and they should be discussed as part of an informed conversation with your provider, during which you weigh all the options. The Thirty-Day Hormone Reset (Chapter 9) provides guidance to determine whether you may want to consider HRT.

The Difference Between Prescription Hormones for HRT and Bio-identical Hormones

Hormone replacement therapy can be a lifesaver for millions of women. But it can also cause problems in the form of side effects—or even be ineffective. Prescription hormones have been around for decades, yet some of those most commonly prescribed have never had their formulas updated!

Conventionally prescribed hormones come only in standard doses. Some of the older ones, such as Premarin (as mentioned, an estrogen formulation made from horse urine), often don't even resemble human estrogen. These prescriptions can be seen as almost foreign substances when they enter our body, creating all kinds of health issues.

Bio-identical hormones, on the other hand, are chemically identical to the structure of our body's own hormones. They need to be made in a compounding pharmacy but they can be tailored for your individual needs, which is particularly useful for people who may have trouble metabolizing certain formulations effectively.

The differences between prescribed hormones and bio-identical hormones have led to controversy. There's a faction of mainstream medical practitioners trying to stop the prescribing of bio-identical hormones. They claim that you can't trust some of the compounding pharmacies. But these naysayers also don't admit to the potential harm that conventional pharmaceutical preparations can cause. Synthroid (levothyroxine sodium), for example, is commonly prescribed for thyroid conditions; it contains gluten, and that very same gluten can trigger symptoms in those with celiac disease or gluten sensitivity.

Some of my patients tell me they will never take conventional medications, limiting themselves to bio-identical formulas. That's not the right attitude, either! Treatments can't be thought of in black-and-white terms. What works for your sister or best friend might not work for you, for instance. Have an open mind and understand that the hormone toolbox is expanding.

Dirty Hormones

A part of the conversation around hormones and hormone balancing is finding the sweet spot where hormones are not too low and not too high and they are being metabolized well, broken down effectively, and utilized by the body.

But when the more toxic or troublesome metabolites of hormones build up, they contribute to many of the hormone symptoms and conditions we have been discussing. In practice, we look for dirty hormones, which include the following:

Estrone: a by-product of estrogen that is stored in the body

17-OH Progesterone: a progesterone metabolite that may mimic androgens

DHT: an androgenic derivative of testosterone that triggers acne and hair loss

Fructosamine: a blood sugar responder that can indicate insulin resistance

C-peptide: an insulin precursor that can indicate insulin resistance prior to an elevated Hgb A1C (blood sugar average over 3 months)

Androstenedione: a metabolite of testosterone that is also androgenic, leading to hair loss and acne

The Hormone Tests You Need

Know Your Numbers

One of the most important steps you can take while assessing your health is to check your hormones with some regularity. The minimum testing is yearly, and ideally it is every six months. If you are going through a shift, the hormones should be checked every three to four months. Checking your hormones is not just about hormones, though; you gain a whole-body snapshot of overall your health and vitality. The hormones are pulling the strings on all aspects of your health as a woman!

I can't stress enough the importance of knowing your numbers. This can be accomplished only with regular testing so the results can be compared over a period of time and any trends and patterns become noticeable. And frequent tests are by far one of the easiest ways for you to assess and monitor your health, so be proactive and catch problems *before* they become chronic or overwhelming. And remember—your hormones fluctuate with your menstrual cycle, so if you are tested at different times within your cycle, your levels will be different; nevertheless, there are clear benchmarks that your numbers should not be above or below. If they are off, these numbers are early warning signs that your body is not where it should be. If they are good, the numbers reinforce that you are making the best choices.

Typically, in Western medicine, there are set markers for routine blood work. Yet those markers sometimes don't work for you. For example, some of my patients with thyroid problems feel great when their TSH is between 1.0 and 2.0; the normal range is 0.8 to 4.0. Then they feel terrible if their range is anywhere above 2.0 or below 1.0. Rather, they need to be tracked consistently to assess their true status.

So, no matter what your age, if you're taking hormones for any kind of treatment, ideally you should be seen at least twice a year—and quarterly, if at all possible. (I know quarterly is inconvenient and often not feasible fiscally.) This is even more important after menopause, when you still need to know what's going on with your body and if it's converting anything into estrogen. We all want to be thriving as we go into this next phase of life—and you certainly don't want surprises to slow you down or stop you in your tracks.

In summary, these testing guidelines are recommended, depending on your hormonal shift:

ROCK STAR (AGES 13-19)

Blood work, pelvic exam/ultrasound every one to two years

HUSTLER (AGES 20-28)

Blood work, pelvic exam/ultrasound annually

SUPERSTAR (AGES 29-38)

Blood work, pelvic exam/ultrasound, breast self exam, thermography yearly

SUPERWOMAN (AGES 39-55)

Blood work, pelvic exam/ultrasound every twelve months, mammogram annually, colonoscopy every five to ten years, thermography annually

COMMANDER (AGES 55+)

Blood work every six months, mammogram and thermography annually, bone scan every five years, colonoscopy every ten years until age seventy-five

Note: These should increase in frequency if you are having any issues or continued symptoms.

Basic Blood Work

The following are my recommendations for basic blood work you need for the tests mentioned in this chapter. All women should have these tests done. If you have a specific or more complex medical condition, further testing should be discussed with your provider. Again, this is basic hormone testing that is still not being done regularly on most women today.

Hormone	Goal Range
DHEA	100–200 μg/dL
Estrogen—estrone (E1)	Never over 150 pg/mL
Estrogen—estradiol (E2)	Never over 200 pg/mL (never under 50 pg/mL unless in menopause and this is goal replacement level)
Insulin, fasting	3–5 μIU/mL
Hgb A1C	5–5.5%
Progesterone	Never less than 0.5 ng/mL (or μg) (also replacement goal)
Testosterone—total	20–40 ng/dL (will be low in menopause but these are hormone replacement goals)
Testosterone—free	1–2 ng/dL
Thyroid TSH	1–2 mIU/L
Thyroid total T3	100–20 ng/dL
Thyroid total T4	5–11.5 μg/dL

Saliva, Adrenal, and Cognitive Testing

In addition to blood work, holistic, integrative, and functional medicine practitioners often suggest tests that evaluate not only *active* levels of hormones and nutrients but also *stored* levels; this gives a better understanding of what the body is doing, not just minute-to-minute but also over time.

Saliva testing. This is often dismissed by Western physicians, but it can provide important information about stored levels of hormones versus active circulating levels. It's another way of looking at how your hormones and metabolism are functioning. I have caught high levels of stored estrogen or testosterone on these lab results, as well as low levels of progesterone that did not match what routine blood work suggested, saving patients' lives from hormone-based diseases. I like saliva testing for more in-depth evaluations of cortisol, estrogen, testosterone, progesterone, and the androgens.

Adrenal testing. It is very difficult to measure cortisol levels in routine lab work—usually only a morning cortisol is valid. Instead, doing a twenty-four-hour cortisol panel can be helpful, and getting levels throughout a day helps pinpoint the stages of adrenal fatigue more accurately. Many of these tests require three to five samples over twenty-four hours to help identify the pattern of adrenal or cortisol secretion that may be causing the symptoms.

Cognitive testing. Chronically overlooked is the state of the brain, even though cognitive health plays into a person's overall health and is heavily influenced by hormones. For patients with cognitive symptoms, such as memory loss, confusion, trouble focusing, or brain fog, I like to use the Gibson Test of Cognitive Skills. It assesses cognitive trends, weaknesses, and key cognitive skills: memory, processing speed, auditory processing, visual processing, logic and reasoning, and word attack skills. There are other surveys and screens doctors use as well.

A more advanced cognitive testing level is a functional MRI, which can show the areas of the brain that might be compromised. This can help if you might have early onset Alzheimer's or dementia through loss of brain volume. If you notice your brain or your cognitive skills shifting, it's time to see a neurologist and demand an MRI, just to be sure.

Imaging Is Hormonal, Too

When I tell my patients that getting a mammogram is hormonal, they look at me like I have said something totally absurd! But it's true. A mammogram or a bone density test isn't just structural—your *hormones* influence what you're seeing in those images. If you tend to store estrogen, then you're going to have a lot of estrogen dominance, and this will show up as dense breasts, fibrocystic breasts, calcified breasts, or breast fibroadenomas.

One extremely important diagnostic imaging test is a *pelvic ultrasound*. You should always request this at your yearly gynecological exam to see what's going on with your reproductive organs. This test is routinely done during pregnancy, but not before or after, and I just don't get it. For example, you may have a thickened endometrial lining, fibroids, ovarian cysts, or a retro- or anteverted uterus—all of which can help connect the dots on your hormone health. I feel strongly that every woman should have routine pelvic ultrasounds to help reassess her hormone health.

Is Genetic Testing Recommended for Hormonal Conditions?

A part of the HRT conversation is understanding your genetic risk for poor hormone detoxification. Genes like MTHFR, COMT, and CYP1B1 can all cause difficulty with estrogen breakdown and metabolism.

The advantage of genetic testing is the ability to use the information and data to plan out what your body does and does not need, and where it may get into trouble. Often, patients see genetic testing as a sentence of some kind, but the fact that you have a genetic predisposition to a condition doesn't mean you're going to develop that condition. When we as medical providers can use genetic testing to educate our patients on what they need and how to individualize their hormone plan, now that's a powerful prescription for healing.

Congratulations! You've made it this far, having completed a crash course in hormones. Review the Hormone Symptom Checklist in Chapter 2 (page 62). Remember, if there are more than five symptoms marked, then, yes, you are dealing with Hormone Hell. See the Appendix for some resources you can use to prepare for your next doctor's appointment. Whether you are a Rock Star or a Commander, Hormone Hell is not only a physical journey—it's an emotional one too.

chapter 4

The Science of Emotions

Breaking news: Your emotions and hormones talk to each other—and together they influence how you feel, think, and even what you will say or do. Trouble.

Here's the thing. Your emotional body—that layer of you that you can't touch, pound on, or measure in blood, saliva, or urine—is controlling your hormones. And your hormones—yes, all the ones you studied in Hormone University (Chapter 3)—are controlling your emotions. The two, with the help of your intellect and will, may meet in the middle, but your body is keeping score; and it's an *emotional, physical, mental, and energetic score.*

The EastWest approach to hormone balancing takes your emotional body into account. What does this mean for all of us? It means that the hurts, disappointments, joys, and anger we have experienced over our years, whether we now are fifteen or fifty, all live within us in our cells. Science is proving this. Did you know that our mitochondrial DNA—the powerhouse of the cells—is where emotions are stored? It is this very DNA that gets handed down, generation after generation. I discussed this in my 2017 TED talk, and it seemed so out-there at the time, but now we know even more: that how we *feel* changes our chemistry, our biology, and of course our hormones. It influences the generations to come. And we, in turn, have been influenced by the seven generations that preceded us.

While science is stumbling, battling this out, I get to see the evidence every day in my practice. I recognize it by applying my EastWest approach to medicine and healing. My patients all have a story—some stories of incredible wins, others of great losses. The feelings reflected in these stories have an energy of their own, which lives in the cells and blocks or aids the flow of energy along a meridian, affecting their *qi*, or overall energy.

This is why I can almost eerily predict how some stories play out. My patients who have experienced loss or divorce hold that grief and anger in their lungs or liver—the key detox organs. Those pathways then get blocked, and guess what sits on the liver meridian? The breasts. So, it is without surprise I often watch a patient go through a painful divorce or career upheaval, only to be diagnosed with an illness or medical condition eighteen months later. Or, I see how a constant worry about a troubled child leads to a digestive issue, because that stress is stored in the gut or spleen meridian, causing cortisol and insulin dysfunction.

And it's not just true of my patients. I have personally experienced this as well, multiple times. The stress and chaos of my childhood home led to my high levels of androgens and insulin, with acne showing up as early as when I was thirteen or fourteen and persisting until I was thirty, when I finally assembled the puzzle pieces. Then, in 2019, my husband had an unexpected heart attack when he was only forty-one; my daughter started her own hormonal swings with mood issues to follow; and I went through some shocking changes, losses, and betrayals at work. It was hit after hit after hit. I was shell-shocked, shaken to my core, and my hormones were sure to tell me. My once-regular periods became heavy and irregular, leaking through pads, tampons, clothes multiple times each month. My belly ballooned from out of nowhere. I was certainly not myself. My body, like those of my patients, was talking to me. Even if I did not have the energy to listen, it was determined to get my attention.

I have had so many patients tell me similar stories. As they navigate their lives and manage their relationships, their loved ones or coworkers tell them the same thing: "You're not yourself."

Of course, there can be many reasons why you are seemingly not yourself. You may be trying to fit in to a new job, move to a new home, care for a newborn with colic, help a friend or family member in crisis, all the time acting as Superwoman to all and bearing the burdens of all their problems. But there is one huge reason for your not being yourself, and it is almost always overlooked by medical professionals.

As you've learned in Chapters 1 through 3, when your hormones are not in balance, your emotions and your mental processing are not in balance either. The world seems dark—much darker than it needs to be. An extreme emotional crisis is waiting to crash your hormones—and a pill can't fix that.

I am sure you know this already; we all know it because we've experienced it. You love your partner or child, and then want them to disappear. Or, you're thinking that something is wrong with them or you, or your relationship. Suddenly you are anxious or depressed or moody or irritable—feelings that magically disappear at some point in your cycle. You're happy one moment, snapping at others the next.

You're able to juggle many tasks and check off those lists, but you're now sobbing hysterically.

Here's the kicker: this all gets amplified in perimenopause and menopause, where the divide widens between the hormones estrogen and progesterone, leading to the hormone depletion of menopause. Jobs are lost, relationships break up, unhealthy habits set in, and you become the very stereotype you always shot down: angry, bitchy, irrational, batty. And the not-so-funny jokes set in about women in perimenopause and menopause.

This is one of the most important points made in this book: *Hormonal shifts or hormonal imbalances are rarely investigated as one of the root causes of emotional issues or mental health conditions. And the impact of trauma, loss, and emotional upheaval is rarely investigated beyond counseling or grief therapy.*

Talk therapy, grief counseling, and finding and healing your inner child is important work, but it's not enough. If you go to a psychiatrist because you're depressed, you'll be asked to describe what is going on in your life that makes you feel that way. There are many causes and variables, of course, but what are the chances this psychiatrist will suggest you get a full medical checkup, with an emphasis on your hormones? I'd say they are pretty close to zero. Instead, you'll leave with a prescription for medication, when what you really need is someone to connect the dots for you. Sadly, that rarely happens. Women—and women's lives—continue to needlessly suffer.

Not on my watch. And not in this book. You have learned so much about hormones already. Now, let's examine the hormone-emotion connection.

The Top Ten Emotions Stored in the Body

How are you, really?

How and what you feel matters. As you'll see in Chapter 5, traditional Chinese medicine (TCM) and Ayurveda connect specific emotions to specific organs and meridians in the body, which also means that every meridian has a correlating emotional association, or a place where that emotion is stored. Your heart hurts with extreme pain or great love. You feel energy flowing when you are in a good place, but have stomach issues when you are anxious. Your throat dries when you cannot express yourself, and your head hurts when there is great tension. We already know there is an emotion-body connection. I am now going to take that one step further and connect it to your hormones.

The following are the ten emotions we most commonly navigate as we journey through life, and each of these emotions has an impact on our physical bodies and hormones. As you read down this list, ask yourself where you are on this emotional spectrum. Which emotions dominate your daily being, your weekdays, or your weekends? Where do you live, emotionally?

JOY/HAPPINESS—Crown

Elation, wonder, joy—the ability to stay in this state of extreme abundance, no matter what life throws at you, is an emotional accomplishment and is consistent with the calling of your seventh and highest chakra. (You will read about chakras in Chapter 5.) This vibrational state allows you to receive direction, guidance, and love from all that surrounds you, and it helps you erect a barrier to negative emotions lower on this list that can take this feeling away.

Are You Depressed?

The Depression Checklist

Depression is a real disease for many women and men, and when it surpasses a feeling and becomes a constant, debilitating experience, a professional medical team is needed. According to the Substance Abuse and Mental Health Services Administration, if these symptoms persist, you may be depressed:

- Sadness
- Loss of interest or pleasure in activities you used to enjoy
- Change in weight
- Difficulty sleeping or oversleeping
- Energy loss
- Feelings of worthlessness
- Thoughts of death or suicide

If you are experiencing these emotions or issues more than one day per week, please see your doctor or a professional to get help.

As you move your hand above your head, think about what that feels like. Is it warm or cold air? Blocked or open? Finding joy in the tiniest elements of your daily life will keep this feeling alive. Of course, the big moments help—that first day on the job you always wanted, reconnecting with your best friend from childhood, getting engaged, having babies—but those milestones are moments and are not forever.

Joy and happiness reduce the cortisol levels, regulate insulin production, and support the hypothalamic–pituitary axis (HPA). Deeper sleep, steady appetite, and more energy become normal rather than stressed. But while it's not easy to get here, it is your ultimate challenge.

Are You Anxious?

The Anxiety Checklist

Most of us today are elevated to some level of anxiety; with the news, the world condition, and the rapid pace at which we all move, anxiety has become a global epidemic. But there's a difference between crippling anxiety and low-grade anxiety. Where do you find yourself?

According to the Substance Abuse and Mental Health Services Administration, if these symptoms persist, you may have anxiety:

- Panic and fear
- Rapid heartbeat
- Shortness of breath
- Trembling
- A strong desire to get away
- Chest pain
- Dizziness

If you experience any of these symptoms more than one day a week, please see a medical professional to start building your toolbox.

LOVE—Heart

Sitting right in the middle of your chest, this fourth chakra organ corresponds to the heart meridian in Chinese medicine, and it is a flow state or an emotional state many of us have and continue to experience. This is not infatuation or possession but, rather, a warmth you can feel in your heart that often is the energy and the motivation to move forward, change, or protect.

We can love our families, children, spouses, and even our work, but the real challenge on this journey is upward: do you love yourself? That warmth should extend to each of us, providing us all with the energy to actually take care of ourselves. What to eat, getting that massage, leaving a toxic relationship—your self-love should motivate you.

In Chinese medicine, when the heart meridian is blocked, there is depression, and when this meridian is overworking, anxiety. Where is your love? Is it directed at yourself? Or to others? Is it too much or too little?

HOPE—Pericardium

Hope lives close to the heart, helping keep the rhythm intact, protecting it to a point, and facilitating love. In a flow state, or on the Journey UP, we are hopeful that challenging situations will work out, even if we are not feeling love. That's why hope is one step down from love and one step up from peace, or neutrality. Hope is the spring, the promise, the place to land when you are navigating around obstacles. If you are not ready for love or to love, or you are not feeling the love, maybe you have hope that you will one day.

PEACE—Circulation/Blood

Peace is the gateway to love and hope. It's a free-flowing state, without obstacles. It's neutral, actually, and not a bad place to land, especially after trauma, disappointment, or even a huge win. I meet so many women (and I may have to include myself in this) for whom the amazing high of an accomplishment soon settles and leaves them searching for the next euphoria.

I think a better plan—one I have actually followed myself—is to move from the highs and the lows to this neutral state, and to stay here for a bit so your body and mind get accustomed to this emotional position, rather than swinging from one extreme to another. Here, the body can rest.

When your blood, or circulation, is flowing, your gut and hormones are nourished and happy, and the cortisol level starts to lower.

ACCEPTANCE—Throat

The throat is the organ of acceptance—of self-acceptance and acceptance by your partners, family, community, and peers. Acceptance leads to self-expression; it's the ability to speak, advocate, and stand up for yourself and for others.

Blockages in this fifth chakra organ are linked to issues concerning acceptance and expression, which in turn influence thyroid regulation. Sounds crazy, but yes, it's all connected.

WORRY—Spleen and Small Intestine

In traditional Chinese medicine, worry impacts the digestive system— specifically, the spleen and small intestine meridians that regulate digestion. My chronic worriers do indeed have gut issues—leaky gut, *Candida* infections, food allergies and intolerances, reflux—you get it. All this gut disruption leads to insulin resistance and high cortisol levels, which can bring about weight gain (particularly belly fat) and fatigue.

FEAR—Kidneys and Bladder

Staying on the Chinese medicine train, we see that the emotion of fear lives in the kidneys and bladder. Fear thus impacts inflammation, the thyroid-adrenal balance, and the fluid and electrolyte balance. Chinese medicine recognizes this and supplies kidney-strengthening tonics and herbs to help release emotions like fear. Its practitioners believe that these emotions are released through chanting, acupuncture, and prayer, for example. In Chapter 9, you will learn how to incorporate an emotional release plan into your Thirty-Day Hormone Reset.

GRIEF—Lungs

Trauma and loss trigger grief, one of the toughest emotions in the world of human experience. In Eastern medicine, this emotion lives in the lungs; for example, grief may cause you to feel like you can't breathe, can't get air. Well, there is a reason for that feeling when we look to Chinese medicine. A deficiency or state of depletion sets in, and hormones like progesterone and estrogen crash. If you are navigating grief, an Eastern medicine provider would assess your hormones, nutrients, and emotional bandwidth—nurturing the patient physically to allow healing in their emotional body.

ANGER—Liver and Gallbladder

With cases of trauma, an emotion preceding grief often is anger. I wish this weren't true, but I have repeatedly witnessed such anger—not the "I got angry because the doctor was late" anger (I know my patients think this) but the deep anger you cannot shake. It is thought this type of anger may stem from a past experience or trauma.

According to traditional Chinese medicine, anger and stress are associated with the liver, and you know by now how important the liver is for hormone balance. When anger is not released, estrogen dominance, thyroid dysfunction, and elevated cortisol take over, and patients don't understand why they are not getting better. Instead, they look at me quizzically when I ask them if they have released their anger.

HATE—Pelvis

The lowest-level emotion, hate is that strong feeling of not liking yourself or another, and it is destructive. Hate leads to self-harm. It serves to block you from finding and experiencing joy or love. And it is a friend to high cortisol levels, leaky gut, and insulin issues.

Hate lives in the pelvis, and many of my patients who are stuck here have issues with their pelvic floor and sexual health.

There's a range of emotions, as you can see, that exists between negative emotions and positive emotions, with the more negative emotions toward the bottom of a ladder and the more positive ones toward the top. The goal is always to lift your emotions and your vibrations to the next level—the Journey UP, discussed in this book—where the highest levels of emotion are love, peace, and happiness. The lowest levels, as you can see, are hate, anger, and fear. Do you live in this lower space? Well, it's time to move up.

But that's not what usually happens. We are hardwired to shift downward, not upward. And our culture in general likes to watch this shift downward rather than the Journey UP. It's like enjoying that accident or a train wreck in a movie, or relishing reality TV. Instead, it's our job to take ownership of the movement of emotion, to consciously build and develop the tools to move upward, to not let the dark voices of past generations and present culture shift us downward, where others have been relegated—expired, cast away, and dismissed.

If we can't make this shift, our bodies will react negatively, starving our cells of oxygen and vitality, and crashing our hormones—all of which leads to disease. To fully understand the scope of this concept, take a look at the chart that follows.

Emotions/Hormones

Emotion	Meridian	Chakra	Hormone Pattern
Joy/happiness	Triple Energizer	Crown	Overall balance/HPA stability
Love	Heart	Heart	Improved stability of all hormones
Hope	Pericardium	Heart	Lowered cortisol, insulin, high oxytocin
Peace	Blood	Triple Energizer	Cortisol, insulin imbalance
Acceptance	Throat	Throat	Thyroid balance
Worry	Spleen/Small Intestine	Solar	Low testosterone, thyroid imbalance
Fear	Kidney/Bladder	Sacral	Low testosterone, thyroid imbalance
Grief	Lungs	Heart	Estrogen depletion, insulin imbalance
Anger	Liver/Gallbladder	Solar/Sacral	Estrogen dominance, progesterone imbalance, testosterone imbalance, high cortisol
Hate	Pelvis	Root	High cortisol, high insulin, testosterone imbalance

The Emotion-Hormone Connection

The emotion-hormone connection is well recognized in Eastern medicine, and as you can see, we all experience these feelings at some point in our lives. But learning to recognize these feelings for what they are and work to shift them is possible—and it can be the difference between just trying to make it and thriving through life.

Cortisol Imbalance

Cortisol may be the ultimate barometer of our emotional health, with its levels rising and falling as we respond and react to our environment. Stress, anger, trauma, and worry all create high-cortisol states, with the body in fight-or-flight mode. In turn, all other hormones react: insulin levels increase, estrogen dominance sets in, and the thyroid tries its hardest to do its job until it crashes.

Regulating your cortisol may be the first place to start when trying to Journey UP—it determines your emotional bandwidth and your ability to climb the ladder of emotions to those that are more positive and uplifting. No wonder mindfulness, breath work, journaling, and so many other modalities are going mainstream; if we want to rise and heal, then we have to bring the cortisol into balance, lest our hormones, and the rest of our body, rebel.

Estrogen Imbalance

When estrogen levels are off, either too low or too high, depression tends to be the dominant symptom. Women feel extremely tired and sluggish. They may find themselves crying, without understanding *why* the tears are falling. The depression can lead to anxiety, as the stressors of life suddenly become too much to manage.

There are two key patterns of estrogen imbalance: estrogen dominance and estrogen depletion. In *estrogen dominance*, the body is unable to break the estrogen down effectively, or it is producing or is exposed to too many environmental estrogens. Sluggish livers, anger and hate, poor diet, chemical overload, and gut dysfunction are all causes of estrogen dominance. Along with this is genetics, which often predict an inability to break estrogen down, as seen in the MTHFR/COMT/CYP1B1 genes. Common symptoms of estrogen dominance include breast tenderness, weight gain, brain fog, fibroids, PCOS, endometriosis, and ovarian cysts.

On the other hand, *low estrogen* or *estrogen depletion* causes weight gain, fatigue, hair loss, wrinkling and skin changes, and bone loss. Grief and trauma can trigger estrogen depletion.

Progesterone Imbalance

Like estrogen, progesterone has a sweet spot. Too much and there are pregnancy-like symptoms: brain fog, heaviness, breast tenderness, belly weight, and bloating. When progesterone is too low, then there are shorter or heavier cycles, palpitations, and anxiety.

Chronic fear and worry trigger low progesterone, and if this pattern continues unchecked, both hormonally and emotionally, the emotional journey spirals down, with anger and hate setting in. I have had couples come in to my practice, and the men are so confused: "I don't know why my wife is so angry all the time. She's mean to everybody. That's not really who she is and I don't know what to do about it."

Sometimes the situation escalates to the point where the couple splits up, especially when that anxiety has turned into rage. This is so upsetting to me that the couples don't realize there's a chemical imbalance at play that likely has worsened existing relationship dynamics. Maybe we should try hormone balancing before divorce? Then therapy? And a peek at the emotional spectrum? Just a thought.

Estrogen and Progesterone Imbalance

Combine an estrogen imbalance with a progesterone imbalance, and you have an altered estrogen:progesterone ratio. What does that mean? More symptoms, more issues with emotional regulation, and lots of cognitive complaints.

What I hear all the time is "I feel stupid. I can't remember anything anymore. I can't focus. I'm not as smart as I used to be. I can't function." This is quickly followed with "I'm just getting old. I *feel* old." And then the hate sets in. Ugh.

Testosterone Imbalance

Testosterone is just as important for women as it is for men. Too much testosterone makes a woman feel aggressive and angry, as if on edge and ready to blow at any moment. You might also feel like you're nagging all the time, smart-mouthing, and being upset and miserable. While acne and hair loss are the physical symptoms of too much testosterone, anger and hate can be the emotional fallout.

Too little testosterone will do the opposite: dampen the libido, cause fatigue and depression, even impact bone health. There is more worry and fear when testosterone levels drop, impacting decisions and movement forward.

Thyroid Imbalance

Okay, by now you are not going to be surprised: the thyroid hormones also need to be in a sweet spot. Too much thyroid—hyperthyroidism—can trigger fear, worry, and overall anxiety. Too little thyroid—hypothyroidism—and we're back to sadness and depression.

Insulin Imbalance

Studies continue to reveal how chronic stress and trauma trigger insulin resistance, raising blood sugar and insulin levels as a response to trauma, grief, anger, fear, and other negative emotions.

This is why after traumatic or repeatedly stressful events, many men and women will experience weight gain, belly fat, or joint pain. In fact, high insulin is associated with inflammation, and I have seen firsthand how expression of autoimmune disease and even cancer show up after one experiences grief, trauma, anger, or deep worry.

Widening Your Emotional Bandwidth

So, I have been talking a lot about the Journey UP, and part of that journey is moving up the emotional ladder, not by avoiding negative emotions or having "toxic positivity" but, rather, by learning to acknowledge emotions for what they are and then building a toolbox to move these emotions through the body, learning to rephrase or rewire them into a more positive form.

That's why recognizing where you are on the emotional ladder is so important. Many of us don't even realize where we are living in our emotional bodies, let alone acknowledge the hormone connection. I challenge you to find your current resting state of emotions and identify which higher emotion you may want to embrace. This is the process of widening your emotional bandwidth, and it is part of the EastWest approach to hormone balancing. It is, to be honest, the secret to good health, success, and finding your purpose and passion. We can't go up if we stay down.

UPWARD SPIRAL

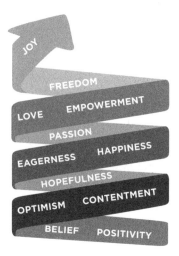

DOWNWARD SPIRAL

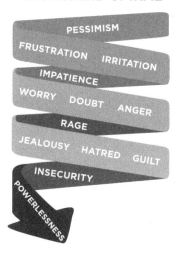

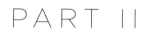

PART II

Superpowered: The EastWest Approach to Hormone Balance

chapter 5

Eastern and Western Healing Modalities

The best method I've found for shifting out of Hormone Hell is to blend the best of Eastern and Western medicines.

Finding your superpowers is easy when you use both Eastern and Western medicine. I learned this personally in my own health journey, and I observe the same results with my patients, day in and day out. When we merge different systems of medicine, we get answers that allow us to connect the dots between our chemistry, our thoughts, our emotions and feelings, and the way we live our lives. I call this the PowerR$_x$ method because, after all, it is leading you to realize your powers.

I know what you are thinking. You just got through the hormone fundamentals at Hormone University, but yes, there is more to learn. Here is the magic. You'll now understand why conventional Western medicine provides some answers—but not all of them—while Eastern medicine brings it all home, completing the puzzle of YOU.

Western Approaches to Healthcare

Conventional Allopathic Medicine, a.k.a. Western Medicine

When most Americans say "I'm going to the doctor," they mean they are going to a practitioner of Western medicine. This is also called conventional, mainstream, standard, orthodox, or allopathic medicine. The category covers MDs and DOs of all specialties, including surgeons, osteopaths, nurses, nurse practitioners, pharmacists, and therapists. And these people identify, diagnose, and treat symptoms and diseases using drugs, radiation, surgery, or a combination of the three.

Western medicine is protocol-driven and science-driven, usually treating one organ or system at a time. This is where the phrase "This is what we always do" comes in, or "This is evidence-based medicine." There is the standard playbook for what to do. If you have thyroid issues, for example, the problem will be treated with medication and/or surgery, but any links to the rest of your body might not be addressed. Think of the Western model as reductionist, meaning that everything—from body parts to body systems, to the mind and heart—is reduced to science, chemistry, and technology.

A reductionist approach to healthcare is not necessarily a bad thing. The treatments of Western medicine can and will save lives. It does an outstanding job for acute care because science, chemistry, and technology can be applied for treatment. If you have an infection, if you break a bone, if you have any kind of emergency or severe illness or disease, Western medicine can often be the quickest and most reliable way to get you better. Civilization itself was transformed for the better when antibiotics, vaccines, anesthesia, and prescription medications became commonplace. New discoveries—thanks to the brilliant minds of researchers, especially in the fields of genetics, the gut microbiome, mental health, organ transplantation, reproductive technology, and rare diseases—are being made all the time.

The problem with Western medicine is that it's sometimes too much a one-size-fits-all methodology and mentality, leaving little room for creative thinking or consideration of the patient as an individual rather than a statistic. As I've mentioned previously, a huge problem for those with hormone issues is that the research and testing of new medications often excludes women, so we suffer the consequences. Or, it fails to differentiate among age, race, or the genetics that influence how hormones work.

When there's not a lot of individualization or personalization of care, hanging your hat on one-dimensional, data-driven evidence (such as standardized blood tests) can result in decisions that don't work for you. In other words, Western medicine takes into account your body's chemistry and biology at a fixed point in time, but it does not account for the meshing of all your body's emotional, mental, spiritual, energetic, and physical factors. The fluidity of our bodies is an Eastern concept, while for Western medicine our bodies are in a fixed state. This is why the EastWest approach to hormone balancing works; it honors the shifting nature of our hormones, and it recognizes that a data point is just one data point; there are so many more data points to understand and link together.

I don't blame the Western doctors. I blame the Western medical school training that pays almost no attention to female hormones outside of pregnancy, that limits the focus on nutrition, and that does not acknowledge the role of toxins in our environment. What do new doctors (and even seasoned ones) do or say? "This is what we always do," and "This is the only way." Or, my favorite, "You're fine."

As we get increasingly more high-tech in medicine, we also get low-touch. Many doctors today don't do physical exams or even touch the patient. Yet there is so much we can learn from a physical exam, from facial diagnostics to thyroid evaluations, gut and liver health, lungs, heart, eyes, ears—should I go on? There is a story told by each of these organs that a discerning provider can use to help put you back into good health.

We have a training issue, and a knowledge gap problem for women's health, for sure. Here's an interesting story regarding this. Back in 2012 or so, my practice was getting a lot of exposure and there was interest from medical residents at the local, well-esteemed academic university. So, we created a preceptorship for them with the university, and their residents were allowed to follow my team at CentreSpringMD. I also lectured the residents on their campus and at local hospitals. This went on for several productive and encouraging years, and we had a good relationship. But out of the blue I received a letter from a dean at the university telling me that they no longer wanted to continue working with me, and that I was to take down any mention of the university from my website. I was shocked, as was the department head I worked with. She investigated to find out what had happened. Apparently, a male doctor had complained about me and the type of medicine I was practicing. One male doctor who had never even set foot in my clinic, one random complaint, and the dean cut the cord. The department head was upset. I was upset. They obviously saw me as a threat.

But I didn't want to fight them, so I just left it alone and continued practicing my kind of medicine. We have expanded from that time to a ten-provider, multi-practice organization that continues to demand future growth. Change is possible. I see it every day.

But we also have a system issue. Physicians who accept medical insurance aren't given enough time with patients, thanks to standard reimbursements; this makes spending enough time with patients unrealistic if you want to keep your practice financially solvent. And don't get me started on the problems inherent to our entire medical system, whereby insurance companies are allowed to make life-altering decisions about treatments they will or will not pay for. Even if you have a good insurance plan, you can be billed for tens of thousands of dollars. The astronomical costs of medical care turn us all away, even when it's desperately needed. My doctors wanted a follow-up MRI on my breasts to make sure everything looked okay, but the bill for doing so was to be $5,000 and the insurance company would be billed a total of $13,000—so of course I would think twice before doing the requested test. (FYI, my husband made me do it, and yes, everything is fine.)

We have a high-tech, high-cost, lifesaving medical system for when patients are in a crisis. But what we don't have is a system that values the uniqueness of *you*. Frustrations with our delivery of medicine has led to the growth of many different medical models and styles of medicine. It is exciting to see this growth, but I often hear the words *holistic, integrative, functional,* and *alternative medicine* all jumbled together, sometimes not even associated with "real doctors."

Integrative Medicine

In my practices, we combine the best of both conventional Western medicine and Eastern medicine, the latter which includes Chinese medicine, Ayurvedic medicine, and many other energy medicine systems. This is, I always say, how medicine should be. We take this knowledge and apply it to each patient, personalizing the treatment. This way is not necessarily rejecting anything from either system; rather, we're looking for treatments from either or both systems that will work and will work safely.

This is the integrative medicine approach, doing what the American Holistic Health Association calls "the art and science of healing that addresses the whole person—body, mind, and spirit." It's why I tell all my patients to keep an open mind, as some have been misdiagnosed earlier or have been gaslighted by Western practitioners and are understandably hostile to that methodology. And this includes patients who have gone the Eastern medicine route exclusively and haven't been handled properly medically, resulting in devastating consequences. This doesn't just happen in America; it occurs all over the world.

My training in integrative medicine was at the University of Arizona, in a fellowship in integrative medicine where its key principles were outlined. For more information about this philosophy, go to integrativemedicine.Arizona.edu.

Functional Medicine

While integrative medicine combines multiple systems of medicine, the rising field of functional medicine takes a more physiological approach, meaning it approaches disease and symptoms by digging deeper into the chemistry, biology, and genetics of a particular issue.

According to the Institute of Functional Medicine (ifm.org), which certifies practitioners in the field, functional medicine "determines how and why illness occurs and restores health by addressing the root causes of disease for each individual." The program views chronic disease as having been caused by a combination of lifestyle choices, environmental factors, and genetic influences and treats it accordingly.

Complementary/Alternative Medicine

According to the National Institutes of Health, "If a non-mainstream approach is used *together with* conventional medicine, it's considered 'complementary.' If a non-mainstream approach is used *in place of* conventional medicine, it's considered 'alternative.'" With this distinction, all Eastern treatments can be considered alternative when used on their own. If, however, your doctor recommends acupuncture along with prescription painkillers, that treatment is considered complementary.

This may seem like splitting hairs, but the real issue is that anyone can take some courses and call themselves an alternative healer. It's up to you to see what kind of training has been done, what accreditation exists, what kind of licensing is afforded, and how much experience the alternative practitioner has had. Many practitioners also have different billing structures, since alternative therapies and Eastern systems of medicine often are not covered by insurance.

Naturopathic Medicine

Naturopathic physicians (NDs) have had rigorous training like medical doctors have, but their focus is on natural, holistic forms of treatment, with nutrition, supplements, herbal and homeopathic formulas, and hands-on treatments like therapeutic massage and acupuncture. They can order conventional lab work, but they can't prescribe conventional medications.

For example, years before she came to see me, one of my patients had been vomiting and had no energy for months. She consulted six different Western specialists, all of whom dismissed her symptoms; one even told her to "start swimming!" She finally consulted an ND, who listened to her symptoms and then told her it was likely she had black mold in her house and had a vitamin D deficiency. Which, much to her shock, it turned out was true. This patient also had *H. pylori*, a stomach infection, without some of the typical symptoms, which the ND was able to find after sophisticated DNA testing. Instead of the typical Western treatment with harsh, side-effect-laden antibiotics, the ND prescribed herbs to kill the pathogens. The herbs took longer to work but were far gentler and had no side effects.

Homeopaths, Herbalists, and Essential Oils

Homeopathy is one of those alternative treatments that's hard to explain, and as a result it is often mocked by many who know little about it. The approach is based on the principle that "like cures like," so highly diluted forms of medicines are prescribed. Homeopaths believe that the *lower* the dose of the medication, the *greater* its effectiveness.

These principles are why homeopathy is often dismissed, but just because we don't understand it doesn't mean there's not something to it. Homeopathy is based on the relationship of vibrational frequencies to our health, as explained by quantum physics—basically, how our own frequencies can dictate and create dis-ease. I have seen homeopathy work firsthand, but I know that it is one of those modalities that is hard to "prove" in the Western scientific model. So, even though I can't say why homeopathy works, I have found it to be helpful for specific symptoms, including belly pain, diarrhea, and headaches—but I don't use homeopathy to treat disease.

Herbalists study the medicinal properties of herbs and plants and how best to mix them to achieve effective treatments. (Many conventional medications, like aspirin, are based on nature's phytochemicals.) Many practitioners of traditional Chinese medicine are skilled herbalists who can give you relief from hormonal symptoms. If you are interested in this kind of approach, though, avoid self-diagnosis and turn to a traditional Chinese practitioner for help. Many herbal formulas are contraindicated with other herbs or prescription medications, and since these supplements aren't FDA-regulated, you need an experienced provider to help you find high-quality products that actually are what they say they are.

Essential oils is another category with many skeptics, mainly because there's a lot of overpromising in claims about oils being able to cure or heal illnesses or diseases—and that can be dangerous for your health. A lot of essential oils are also highly diluted or adulterated, and their quality depends on the original sourcing of the plants from which they are made.

On the other hand, pure essential oils distilled from plants do have properties that are effective. They can directly impact the hypothalamus, your immune system, and/or your lymphatic system as well as your hormones. They smell wonderful in a bath, put into a diffuser, or added to a carrier oil or lotion for body and hair treatments. Some oils, like rosemary, have been rigorously tested by mainstream scientists, and they do have an immediate effect on the limbic system, which controls your emotional response, so they can make you *feel* better. That is, when inhaled, rosemary essential oil has been shown to invigorate the brain, while lavender oil has a calming effect. Many of the citrus oils are great for a quick wake-up, and tea tree oil can often help control yeast and fungal infections.

The best way to use essential oils is as a supportive adjunct to your overall treatment and an aromatic way to boost your wellness plan. Have fun experimenting with different blends and see which ones are effective for your condition. If you have menstrual cramps, for example, try using a roller-ball applicator to spread an essential oil blend directly on your abdomen to help ease the pain. Smelling something delightful or invigorating can at the very least improve your mood and may well alleviate some of your symptoms by acting on the limbic system in your brain.

Essential Oils for Added Support

In our practice at CentreSpringMD, we incorporate essential oils into our patients' treatment plans as added support. The chart below lists my favorite essential oils that, in my experience with patients, can work in concert with a happy hormone plan to help bring about symptom relief and general relaxation.

Essential Oil	Hormone Pattern
Bergamot	Can help reduce cortisol
Cinnamon	Can help relieve PMS symptoms, especially menstrual cramps
Citrus (lemon, orange)	Can support testosterone and libido
Clary sage	Can help reduce cortisol, improve thyroid health, and relieve PMS symptoms, especially menstrual cramps
Fennel	Can help support estrogen and prolactin
Frankincense	Can help provide thyroid support, cortisol balance
Geranium	Can support estrogen
Lavender	Can help relieve estrogen dominance and PMS symptoms, especially menstrual cramps
Rose	Can help to balance testosterone and androgens, provide PMS relief
Rosemary	Can help relieve estrogen dominance
Thyme	Can support progesterone
Vitex	Can support estrogen and progesterone balance and help reduce prolactin
Ylang ylang	Can support testosterone and libido

Eastern Approaches to Healthcare

Ayurveda

Created in India over 5,000 years ago, *Ayurveda* means "the science of life." Since it has been used successfully for so long, believe me when I say how helpful it can be in the diagnosis and treatment of hormonal issues.

Doshas

The central tenet of Ayurveda is that there are three main energies or personality types, or *doshas*, as well as their combinations. Your energy level, emotional makeup, and hormonal aspects can be predicted with each type of dosha:

- Vata—Often described as thin, wiry, or lanky, Vatas are dominated by the air element and prone to dry skin or hair.
- Pitta—Of medium build and athletic, Pittas are associated with fire. They tend to generate and create more heat, often resulting in digestive issues.
- Kapha—With a larger, more heavy-set build, Kaphas have slower metabolism, thick hair and skin, and a tendency to gain weight.

In addition, each dosha has an element symbolizing its primary energy:

- Air/wind—associated with Vata
- Fire—associated with Pitta
- Earth—associated with Kapha

Air/fire—associated with Vata-Pitta

Earth/air—associated with Vata-Kapha

We all have a dominant dosha; very few people are purely one type. Most of us have elements of all three, but one type is usually dominant. A central principle of Ayurvedic philosophy is the recognition that we are fluid creatures. What you need in one season of your life may differ entirely in a later season. You may always have your dominant energy or dosha, but it can shift through the decades and in response to the stressors, wins, and joys of life. Ayurveda recognizes hormone shifts and aims to provide prescriptive solutions for each of these shifts.

For this reason, Ayurvedic practitioners reassess their patients at every visit, using tongue, face, and pulse diagnoses. They understand that the fluidity of the body means that checking in with yourself is necessary. If we apply these principles today, we would all know our numbers, including hormone levels and optimal nutritional needs through each hormone shift.

There are many tools available to help identify your dosha. The chart that follows is a tool I have used, and it's fairly simple. Place a check mark at each symptom you have. The column with the most checks is your dominant or primary dosha. The one with the next most checks will be your secondary dosha.

Find Your Dosha

	Vata (air)	Pitta (fire)	Kapha (earth)	
Body frame	Long and lean	Moderate	Substantial	
Body weight	Tends to be underweight	Tends to be moderate	Tends to be overweight	
Skin	Dry, rough, cold, thin	Soft, warm, fair, moles and freckles, flushes easily	Oily, thick, cool, pale	

	Vata (air)	Pitta (fire)	Kapha (earth)	
Hair	Dry, rough, brittle, curly or kinky, coarse, light brown	Thin, fine, straight, light-colored, early gray, balding	Thick, oily, wavy, dark brown or black	
Teeth	Irregular, protruding, crooked, thin gums, tendency to tooth decay	Regular, moderate, soft gums, yellowish	Big, white, strong, healthy	
Eyes	Small, darting, brown	Moderate, sharp, intense, greenish	Blue, big, caring, thick eyelashes	
Lips	Thin	Moderate, red	Full, pale	
Neck	Long and thin	Moderate	Short and thick	
Joints	Dry, cracking, cold, bony	Moderate	Well lubricated, large, not visible	
Musculature	Slight and stiff, tendony	Medium, flexible	Firm, stout	
Appetite	Variable, scanty, can miss a meal without noticing it	Good, excessive, gets hangry (hungry and angry) if a meal is missed	Low but steady	
Thirst	Variable	Excessive	Steady	
Sweating	Variable to none	Excessive, odorous	Moderate to none, no odor	
Sleep	Wakes easily, difficult to fall asleep	Falls asleep easily, stays asleep, has difficulty sleeping in warm weather	Sleeps long and deep, has difficulty waking up	
Elimination	Irregular, dry, hard, tends to constipation	Regular, loose, soft, tends to diarrhea	Slow, regular, oily	
Physical activity	Fast and very active	Moderate and competitive	Lethargic and slow	

	Vata (air)	Pitta (fire)	Kapha (earth)	
Dreams	Often fearful, flying, running, jumping, dancing	Often fiery, passionate, angry, violent	Often calm, romantic, watery, of relationships	
Emotions	Unpredictable, anxious, insecure	Irritable, jealous, blaming, judgmental, angry, critical	Calm, quiet, loving	
Mind	Restless, active	Aggressive, intelligent, intense	Calm	
Faith	Changeable	Determined, can be fanatical	Steadfast	
Memory	Recent good, long-term poor	Sharp	Slow but steadfast	
Interests	Creating, running, dancing, talking	Competitive sports, debate, politics	Family and social gatherings, cooking, collecting	
Finances	Poor, spends money on cheaply made items	Moderate, spends money on well-made items	Rich, saves well	
Achieving goals	Easily interrupted and distracted	Focused, driven, production-oriented	Works slowly and steadily	
Relationships	Has many casual acquaintances	Has intense relationships	Has loyal, long-term relationships	
Weather	Averse to cold, windy weather	Averse to hot weather	Averse to cold, damp weather	
Reaction to stress	Excites easily, flies apart in all directions	Rises to the challenge	Rarely gets stressed, plods along	
Shows affection	With words	With gifts	With touch	
	TOTAL VATA:	TOTAL PITTA:	TOTAL KAPHA:	

Chakras

If you've ever done yoga, you will be familiar with chakras, the seven points of spiritual powers or energy centers in your body. Each chakra has a different form of energy, called *prana*, or life energy. Since chakras are connected to your psychological, emotional, and spiritual well-being, when one or more chakras gets blocked, the prana cannot flow and health issues can result. (This is similar to the notion of *qi* and meridians in traditional Chinese medicine.) The chakras are all inter-related, and their goal is to help us grow in our spiritual journey until we reach the highest chakra.

The Seven Chakras

Chakra	Meaning
Crown	Spirituality
Third Eye	Mental focus, clarity, and intelligence
Throat	Communication
Heart	Love
Solar plexus	Confidence and control
Sacral	Connection and acceptance
Root	Foundation and being grounded

Chakras Through the Years

Why do we need to talk of chakras and energy? Well, simply put, the chakras are a part of our spiritual Journey UP as we age. Each phase of life is about strengthening and solidifying at least one of the seven chakras. The following shows how the chakras apply to the five key hormone shifts.

Rock Stars and Hustlers

The Root/Sacral/Solar Plexus chakra is all about stability and foundation. For Rock Stars and Hustlers, building a foundation for careers, relationships, and a healthy home is a driving force.

Superstars

You move up into the Heart chakra as you get into your thirties and become a Superstar. Relationships and community start becoming more important. Caring for others, rather than yourself, starts to take over a bit. Keeping the Heart chakra open and expressive can be a challenge for my Superstars as they start to get overwhelmed with responsibilities.

Superwomen

While in your Superwoman forties, you continue upward, working into the Throat space or fifth chakra, which is about communication. This is where women finally come into their own, able to advocate for themselves, speak their truths, and gain clarity about what they really want.

Commanders

I call this the coronation, when the Crown chakra becomes more active, along with the Third Eye. This leads to greater connection with our spiritual and energetic bodies, and where we have full expression of our goals, desires, and purpose. As we literally rise into these chakras, we stop giving our power away and start making decisions that are congruent with our purpose.

Using Ayurveda for Diagnosis

In India, Ayurvedic training can be as rigorous as Western medical school, and practitioners must do an internship and have a certain number of training hours before they are licensed.

Thanks to my training and years of experience, and because the doshas have innate physical attributes and general principles, I can pretty much always tell which one a new patient is the minute she comes into the exam room and starts describing her symptoms. These physical markers, along with extensive Ayurvedic questionnaires that patients fill out, allow me to start formulating a diagnosis quickly, and then I back it up with lab results to validate my initial impressions.

Each dosha has specific needs and hormone patterns. For instance, I know that Vatas are prone to adrenal and cortisol issues, and often need more healthy fats, protein, and warmer foods. For example, oiling (massaging the scalp or body with warmed sesame or mustard oil) was considered essential for Vatas, so ghee (clarified butter) became a necessary fat for nourishment and replenishment. Pittas (I'm partly one) are prone to thyroid, insulin, and cortisol issues because we tend to *go, go, go, go, go*. Our cortisol levels get out of control and drain the thyroid, and that in turn affects insulin regulation. Kaphas prefer a slower pace, tend to have insulin and estrogen-dominance issues, and are prone to fibroids, heavy periods, and abdominal weight gain. They also need more fiber, more plant-based foods, and less saturated fat and animal protein in their diets.

Now, this has been, as you can see, a two-second download on doshas. There is so much more rich history and prescriptive information in Ayurveda to help keep doshas balanced. So, here's a cheat sheet for the most common disorders for each dosha:

Vata: Thyroid, adrenal dysfunction, cortisol
Pitta: Cortisol, thyroid, progesterone
Kapha: Insulin resistance, estrogen dominance

Ayurvedic treatments follow on the following two steps:
1. *Observation and analysis.* A practitioner looks closely at your body, especially your face and tongue, then listens to your pulse to

identify your dominant dosha and what combination you might be. The lifestyle-evaluation questionnaire also pinpoints issues.

2. *Treatments.* The standard protocol is to address food, mind, body, and supplements. Your practitioner will first recommend changes to your diet, if needed. Next come recommendations for stress relief and ways to improve energy and sleep. Then, body treatments are suggested to relax your nervous system. (Two of my favorite treatments are the super-calming and relaxing *shirodhara*, whereby heated oil is poured over your forehead, accessing the Third Eye or sixth chakra, and *abhyanga* (the Sanskrit word translated as both "oil" and "love"), a fifteen- to twenty-minute self-massage technique that is also extremely calming, hydrates your skin, and even helps your hair grow. If you need an added boost, herbal-based supplements can be recommended, and they are extremely potent and helpful.

Here's an example: me! According to the standard definition of celiac disease, I don't have it and it wouldn't show up on a biopsy. But like many Pittas, I was really suffering with so many symptoms of celiac disease and gluten sensitivity, including joint pain, rashes on my arms known as keratosis pilaris, hair loss, and thyroid issues, that something had to be done. (I think we need to change the definition of celiac disease, as so many people have symptoms and are suffering.) I am a testament to how a simple diet shift can change everything. I started removing gluten from my diet, added nutrients like B vitamins and iodine, added probiotics for improved gut health, and took a low-dose thyroid hormone. Pittas like me benefit from a gluten-free, dairy-free diet that is bolstered by digestive enzymes and probiotics. Sometimes this dietary shift alone is enough to make a huge improvement in hormone levels, as it did for me. The changes didn't happen instantly; it took time—a solid six months to a year—to see marked improvement. But once that happened, the solution was incredibly powerful, and I have not looked back since.

I show you how to incorporate doshas and chakras into the Thirty-Day Hormone Reset (Chapter 9) to bring you into full balance and address the shifts that are part of your health journey.

Honor Your Energy

I had a fascinating conversation with one of my lead nurses recently. She's an LPN, an amazing woman and skilled worker. She was trying to get her RN degree, but she has Hashimoto's disease and tires easily. When she got Covid, she was knocked down entirely.

"I'm so frustrated," she told me. "I have no energy after working to even open my textbooks or do anything. And here's my sister who has two kids, she's going back to school, she's doing all this other stuff, and she seems fine, you know? It's not fair!"

"Well, according to Chinese and Ayurvedic medicine, we're all gifted with a certain amount of energy," I explained. "It's like this little package that we're born with. So, what's actually not fair for you is to compare yourself to your sister, because you're walking through life with a different set of tools, different energy levels, and a different makeup. Please don't beat yourself up! Let's honor the energy you've been given, and do our best to build you up."

By balancing her thyroid, improving her digestive health, and adding the missing nutrients in her diet, her energy soared—and she now has more bandwidth to do the things she always wanted to do, while still honoring the boundaries she needs set for herself.

Traditional Chinese Medicine

Traditional Chinese medicine (TCM) is similar to Ayurveda in its focus on the movement of energy within the body. Ideally, its methods are used to stop disease *before* it occurs, so it is more prophylactic than Western modalities. TCM is also holistic in its view of the body, as a person's emotional makeup and physical needs are interrelated, one affecting the other in a masterful symphony.

The Concepts of Meridians, *Qi*, and Yin and Yang

Meridians

Traditional Chinese medicine believes that there are twelve main channels, or meridians, of energy, or *qi*, that govern the body and its functions. Think of your meridians as highways connecting your blood to your organs and tissues. The meridians exist in corresponding yin-yang pairs; acupuncture is the attempt to move energy that is in blocked meridians and may be leading to disease.

The Twelve Meridians

Meridian/Organ	Emotional Connection	Physical Connection
Bladder	Frustration, poor decision-making	Bladder issues, inflammation
Gallbladder	Anger, decision-making	Headaches, migraines, trouble digesting fat
Heart	Depression	Cardiovascular disease
Kidney	Fear	Kidney issues, hormone balance
Large Intestine	Sadness	Microbial imbalance, digestive issues
Liver	Anger	Detoxification, hormones, insulin

Meridian/Organ	Emotional Connection	Physical Connection
Lung	Grief	Poor detoxification, asthma
Pericardium	Anxiety, mental health	Cardiovascular disease, shortness of breath
Small Intestine	Shame, sadness	Microbial imbalance, digestive issues
Spleen	Worry	Digestion, breakdown of foods and nutrients
Stomach	Anxiety, worry	Acid reflux, bloating
Triple Warmer*	Arrogance	Overall mental health, referred to as *shen* in Chinese medicine

This is the meridian that controls the fight-flight-or-freeze response to stressful situations, and it runs down the center of the body.

Qi

Qi (pronounced CHEE) is the life energy or life force you're born with. It runs along your meridians in an electrical circuit. As your health circumstances change, *qi* can be replenished or depleted; when you're out of balance, it becomes blocked, and this can create disease.

Yin/Yang

The concept of yin/yang is that there are harmonious yet opposing forces meant to balance each other, and this balance is responsible for the quality of your *qi*. Yin is the nurturing female energy; yang is the more aggressive male energy. A perfect balance of the two is the ultimate goal.

Using TCM for Diagnosis

Traditional Chinese medicine is all about making sure your *qi* is moving smoothly. If it's disrupted, the root cause needs to be determined. As with Ayurveda, TCM treatments focus on the following:

Observation and analysis. A practitioner first listens carefully to your pulse, then examines your tongue. For example, a red tongue with cracks and little to no coating shows a yin deficiency, and symptoms are likely to include fatigue, anxiety, and brain fog. The color/skin tint, condition, and texture of specific areas of your face, as well as your eyes, are also examined, as they correspond to the health status of various organs. An acne breakout between your eyebrows, for instance, signifies liver toxicity and hormonal imbalance; dark circles under your eyes often indicate a kidney imbalance.

Face Diagnosis

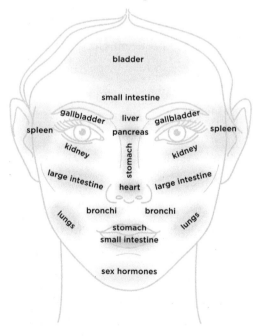

Tongue Diagnosis

Things to look for: size, coating, shape, color, cracks

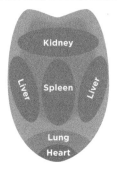

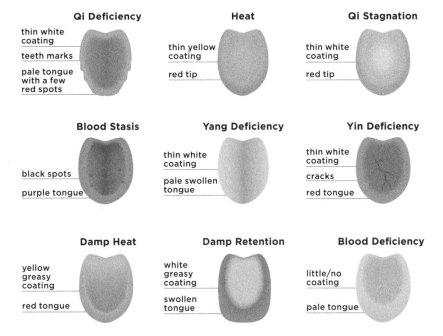

Qi Deficiency

thin white coating

teeth marks

pale tongue with a few red spots

Heat

thin yellow coating

red tip

Qi Stagnation

thin white coating

red tip

Blood Stasis

black spots

purple tongue

Yang Deficiency

thin white coating

pale swollen tongue

Yin Deficiency

thin white coating

cracks

red tongue

Damp Heat

yellow greasy coating

red tongue

Damp Retention

white greasy coating

swollen tongue

Blood Deficiency

little/no coating

pale tongue

Treatments. One of the most powerful treatments in traditional Chinese medicine is acupuncture, whereby superfine needles are inserted at different points in your meridians to unblock the stuck *qi*. As the energy improves and the *qi* is unblocked, the spot will become red and hot—indicating increased blood flow to the damaged area. That redness, thus, is a sign that energy is beginning to move, and with repetition, the meridian flow improves.

Acupuncture is sometimes aided by *moxibustion*, whereby aromatic herbs are heated up over the acupuncture points. *Cupping*, which involves placing small suction cups over particular points, usually on the back, for several minutes, helps detox the body and move the *qi* around. Finally, specific foods and/or herbal supplements are recommended to eat or to avoid, as different items possess different healing properties to balance your yin/yang and open up your meridians.

Using TCM for Hormonal Issues

Hormone balance in traditional Chinese medicine is achieved by strengthening the gut and the liver. These two organs are responsible for how dramatic or how gentle your hormone shifts may be. A healthy, balanced gut and a well-functioning liver create *qi*, or energy. Time and investment in these two organs and the meridian systems allow for minimal hormone replacement, and the hormones often balance themselves.

Also, TCM divides the phases of a woman's life into seven main cycles, or "changes in essence." Keep in mind that these cycles were described when women did not live past sixty years, so now we can add years to each phase. As traditionally written, these phases include the following:

Birth: age 7
Puberty starts: ages 7–14
Full puberty and transition to womanhood: ages 14–21
Most fertile years: ages 21–28
Family and career building: ages 28–35
More family and career building, with added responsibilities and
    the beginning of perimenopause: ages 35–42

Perimenopause: ages 42–49

Completion of "aging" and transition from perimenopause to menopause and your new identity as an elder in the community: ages 49–56+

Hormone balancing in TCM varies according to each cycle and each phase of a woman's life. It combines diet, herbs, exercise, and sleep as prescriptive ways to balance hormones.

Merging Elements of Eastern and Western Medicines

This is where the magic happens; it's where we can connect the dots on emotional health, energy, and body chemistry. Here is where the elements of all parts of our bodies—energetic, emotional, spiritual, physical, and mental—come together to form an expanded toolbox that aids us on our Journey UP.

Merging these systems of medicine is what my team and I have done in our practice for over thirteen years. We know this method works—that's why our approach to hormone balance uses terms like *gut-liver cleanup, detoxification, emotional release,* and *full-body rehab.* By methodically merging a patient's Chinese medicine diagnosis with their Ayurvedic one, and pairing it to lab tests that explore hormone, gut, and nutrient status while ruling out inflammation, poor detoxification genetics, and family health risks, we can make your hormones become your superpower.

Remember, your health is a journey, not a pit stop; when we choose the long game, that's the ultimate win. Quick fixes are just that— temporary and expensive. Realize, too, that a lot of Western medicine is 100 percent triage—the emergency room approach. As in, "Okay, here's the problem. Let's give you an immediate solution. You're better? Great. Stick with the plan. Goodbye." And then come the side effects, the health plateaus are reached, and the secondary conditions and symptoms set in because the root causes, the origins, of the issues were never addressed.

My goal here is to move you beyond that symptom-only approach. Yes, of course you want to get the immediate situation under control. But at the same time you have to build a foundation for good health. This foundation becomes your soul's home, ready to do the work for you that it was meant to do.

Bear in mind that the payoffs from employing your integrative and holistic toolbox are not quick, but they are long-lasting and life-changing. I get to see this in my practice everyday. The merger of Eastern and Western medicine takes you on a journey to your highest self, helping you unlock your superpowers and find your life's mission or purpose.

EastWest Medicine in Practice

I have to be perfectly honest. It took me years of hard work, advanced education, research, and trial and error to develop my system combining the best of Western and Eastern philosophies—what I have been calling the Power R_x approach to hormone balancing. In short, I identify the Ayurvedic dosha and chakra weakness, use TCM to find the meridian imbalance, complete a detailed medical history, order lab tests, and then evaluate all that information to personalize my patients' health plans.

What I often hear from new patients is "Well, my doctor checked my levels, but they said they don't matter because they didn't know where I was in my cycle." I push back on that: There *are* some absolutes that women need in order to feel good. For example, no woman feels good when her progesterone level is under 0.5. No woman feels good when her estrogen level is starting to go below 50.0. You can see how these blanket guidelines don't work for everyone—and make me angry.

These assumptions are one of the reasons all women currently get the same treatment for hormone imbalances or replacement, regardless of personal medical history—as I've mentioned, it's a very Western medicine approach. Our genetics, stressors, gut, and liver health—oh, yes, and nutrition and toxic load—are all different. We each have a unique health fingerprint. So, when my patients ask about hormones, I tell them it's not so much that a particular hormone is bad—a big worry for those who have a family history of estrogen-based breast cancers—but how their bodies are going to detox or break the hormone down. If you have a really weak gut, a toxic liver, or high stress levels and your regular physician gives you a standard prescription of estrogen, progesterone, and testosterone, then, yes, that stuff is going to get stored. And if it gets stored, it's going to activate genetics that probably need to be left alone. I don't want this to happen to my patients, so I try a subtler approach for those who need hormone replacement, as explained in the next section.

Other Treatments I Prescribe

Your gut and your diet are always the starting points, because so much of the hormone story begins here. I learned this hard way because, as part Pitta, I naturally have a lot of digestive fire, leading to digestive problems. I have learned that I need to be on a diet that is anti-inflammatory—low, for example, in gluten and dairy. Otherwise, my gut and liver are overburdened, which triggers thyroid and insulin imbalances.

Next up is a look at any nutrient deficiencies, chronic viruses, and toxicity. So many women have the Epstein-Barr virus or Lyme disease, either of which reactivates when the immune system is weak, or they are exposed to mold (especially in warmer climates like that in the U.S. South, where I live) that wears down the immune system and triggers overgrowth of yeast in the gut, which then triggers hormone issues. Detailed laboratory testing often reveals these issues.

And then there is energy testing, which alerts my attention to issues that lab tests don't reveal or that preemptively identifies vulnerabilities that become obvious on lab work six months later. These energy evaluations are an essential tool in merging the Eastern and Western medicines, helping us assemble the pieces of the puzzle that make up our multidimensional bodies. The physical, emotional, spiritual, and energetic aspects of our bodies are always interconnected, influencing one another. So I ask what emotions are at play; what systems are weak—but not weak enough to show up in lab work; and where we should head as we begin the healing journey. These questions are an incredible tool I use in educating my patients on where they stand and how they can create their personal hormone symphony.

This methodology is essential to the Journey UP, expanding my patients' vitality and helping them climb to grasp their highest powers. Merging the elements of different medicines has worked in my practice for years, helping 30,000 patients. I can't wait to make it work for you.

chapter 6

The Gut-Hormone Connection

Your gut is ground zero for your health. It processes your food. It gets rid of waste. It produces neurotransmitters. It fights off toxins. And it plays a pivotal role in hormone balance.

This is one of the primary reasons I am such a big proponent of merging Eastern and Western medical treatments to achieve happy hormones. Chinese medicine and Ayurveda have for thousands of years linked the state of the gut and digestive health with how the body metabolizes and uses hormones. With the advent of twentieth-century technology, like blood work and other advanced testing that reconfirms their concepts, we now take their contributions for granted. They treated hormonal issues by addressing the patterns they saw when the meridians were stuck, *qi* was low, or prana (the word for the life force) was depleted.

They knew, for example, that spleen meridian issues would result in too much dampness, which would change blood sugar levels. Or, that kidney meridian imbalances would block hormone production, since *qi* would be dissipated. Thyroid disorders were linked to the liver and kidney, while estrogen dominance was a pattern common to those with liver stagnation. But central to their hormone dialogue was the status of the gut. While the spleen meridian regulated digestion and dampness, the small intestine meridian mirrored the microbiome, and too much Pitta triggered heat or excessive digestive fire. They were able to identify a leaky gut or compromised immune system using their ancient methodology. And this is where a plan for hormone balancing was begun.

How often do we make this connection in conventional medicine? Bloating, constipation, diarrhea, and reflux live in the world of gastrointestinal issues, but they are in no way thought to be linked to stored estrogen, the thyroid, progesterone levels, or insulin. In Western medicine, the answer for any GI issue is a prescription for medication to manage the symptoms only, when what is needed is a referral to an endocrinologist or gynecologist for a hormone discussion.

Let's take a look at the patterns of hormone imbalances and digestive health that likely appear.

Gut Issue	Hormone Pattern
Constipation	Estrogen dominance, high insulin
Diarrhea	Low progesterone, sluggish thyroid
Bloating	Thyroid disorders, high or low estrogen, high or low progesterone
Reflux	High progesterone, low estrogen, low testosterone

These patterns were never discussed or reviewed in my medical school education and training; instead, I learned about them by studying Chinese and Ayurvedic medicine and marrying this information to the lab values of my patients. The merger of these different systems of medicine expanded my hormone-treatment toolbox, allowing patients to get better before we even touched an actual hormone. And I realized that the language used to describe certain energy patterns in Chinese medicine and Ayurveda accurately reflected many of the hormone imbalances we identify today through blood work and testing. Let's take a closer look at the various terms for particular gut–hormone conditions.

Meridian Pattern	Ayurvedic Pattern	Gut Issue	Hormone Imbalance
Spleen deficiency	Kapha	Bloating/ constipation	High insulin
Liver stagnation	Pitta	Diarrhea/IBS	Estrogen dominance
Liver yin deficiency	Vata	Bloating/IBS	Low progesterone, low estradiol
Liver-kidney deficiency	Vata/Pitta	Constipation/ reflux	Thyroid disorders
Kidney meridian deficiency	Vata	Bloating	Low estradiol, progesterone, thyroid disorders

Gut Smarts Quiz

In 2014, I wrote the book *The 21-Day Belly Fix* at a time when information about the microbiome was exploding. Here is a mini quiz to help you identify if you have a gut problem, not a just a hormone problem. Answer True (T) or False (F) to each question.

1. I have a bowel movement daily. T F
2. When I use the bathroom, the stool is formed and I feel I have emptied completely. T F
3. I don't experience abdominal pain after eating. T F
4. I rarely have reflux or heartburn. T F

5. I am able to eat and tolerate a wide variety of foods.   T F
6. I don't have skin rashes.   T F
7. I don't have joint pain.   T F
8. I rarely experience bloating.   T F
9. My tongue is red, not coated.   T F
10. My complexion is clear, without unusual redness or puffiness.   T F

If you answered False to more than four questions, your gut may be at the root of many of your symptoms and is likely the factor driving your hormone imbalances.

Hopefully these examples convince you of the gut-hormone connection and how we have to address the gut to balance your hormones.

The Hormone Factory in Your Gut

There are the four main components of gut health that can impact your hormones:

1. Leaky gut
2. Microbial balance—the microbiome
3. Fat malabsorption
4. Poor nutrient quality and quantity

Let's take a look at each of these. And yes, there is a quiz at the end. . . .

Leaky Gut Syndrome

Leaky gut is a term used commonly today, but it is still much debated and often dismissed by the conventional medical community. Leaky gut is, in essence, intestinal malabsorption, whereby the gut lining is no longer intact and healthy, creating a state of low-grade chronic inflammation. This inflammation, in turn, leads to microbial and nutritional shifts that directly impact hormone production. Fortunately, ongoing research has tied gut health to hormone imbalances. These are patterns I see in practice, as well.

There are many Western physicians, even gastroenterologists, who downplay the notion of a leaky gut. If pressed, they might grudgingly call it "increased intestinal permeability" or "malabsorption." I guess *leaky gut* sounds a bit too descriptive for them, but I think it's the perfect term for a legitimate phenomenon that should not be ignored. In fact, it's safe to say that *everyone* has a leaky gut—it just depends on how severe it is.

The lining of the intestine is loaded with hairlike projections called *villi*, which are part of the system that enables digestible nutrients from your food to move along and be absorbed into your bloodstream, then taken to the cells that need them to function. In addition, what connects the intestinal cells to each other are microscopic meshlike structures called *tight junctions*—rather like grout connects your bathroom tiles together. When the gut is healthy, there are no holes or spaces, and all your nutrients pass along the intestines as intended.

So, here's where problems arise. These nutrients have to pass from the villi through your intestinal walls into the bloodstream—and these walls are only one cell-layer thick. Not only does this ridiculously thin layer have to allow the nutrients to pass through, but it also has to prevent toxic invaders from getting in. The human body is a marvel in so many ways, but intestinal permeability is a physiological problem always waiting to happen. When the tight junctions aren't tight enough, breaches both in and out of the intestines start to form. Your gut is literally leaking. Think of a screen door. When working properly, it allows fresh air to pass through it and keeps bugs out. But if there are tears in the screen, bugs and debris will be able go in and out as they please.

The end result? *Inflammation.* Inflammation that leads not only to decreased hormone production but also to disease, as well as to development of autoimmune conditions, cognitive impairments, skin issues, and weight gain. Inflammation also causes systemic stress in the body, leading to overproduction of cortisol, which can then trigger anxiety and deplete the immune system. And almost 95 percent of the neurotransmitters, including serotonin, dopamine, and GABA (gamma-aminobutyric acid), are made in the gut; this directly impacts mood and sleep. No surprise, then, that a leaky gut is often at the root of problems of anxiety, depression, OCD, brain fog, and many other mental health conditions.

Leaky gut is also responsible for nutritional deficiencies. When that screen door is torn, well, there go your nutrients. All that effort to eat well and clean is undermined by a leaky gut. Absorption of the nutrients essential for hormones is blocked, leading to and accelerating hormone imbalances.

Triggers for a Leaky Gut

What can trigger a leaky gut? It's almost always a combination of factors—what I often refer to as the "tipping point in response to a cumulative load." In fact, in my practice I am always looking at patterns of three: the three hits in combination that caused the leaky gut. Everyone's story is individual, but are a few common patterns are:

- Processed/refined foods + stress + poor sleep
- Medications + high toxic load + genetics
- Genetics + inflammation + stress

- Virus + processed foods+ stress
- Insect bite + medication + genetics
- Food intolerances + stress + poor sleep
- Sugar + stress + genetics

How to Test for Leaky Gut

Here is the good news: you can test for a leaky gut and you can heal a leaky gut. Testing methods and research are catching up with what we see in practice. Here are a few current ways to test for leaky gut:

- Stool tests for fecal fats, fecal elastase, zonulin
- Blood tests for nutritional deficiencies, often a sign of leaky gut
- Blood tests for immunoglobulins
- Lactoferrin levels
- Breath tests for mannitol, lactulose
- Blood tests for inflammation markers ESR, CRP, homocysteine

If all roads point to a leaky gut, my Thirty-Day Hormone Reset (Chapter 9) will help get your gut back on track.

Why Your Microbiome Matters

The gut has a vast community of *100 trillion* microbes. These are tiny bacteria that live in your gut, doing the work of assimilating, digesting, absorbing, and transporting nutrients. There are roughly the same number of bacteria in a milliliter of stool as there are stars in the Milky Way—how amazing is that?

Even more astonishing, a woman weighing 150 pounds will have a microbiome weighing 2.5 pounds. That's a lot of bugs—but they are all needed to keep us healthy and to keep our hormones balanced. This is what your microbiome is meant to do:

- Make and process your hormones
- Produce acids to help digest your food
- Help break down certain B vitamins
- Reduce inflammation in your gut
- Help stimulate your immune system
- Rev up your metabolism

And when we turn the spotlight on hormones, check out the gut bacteria–hormone connection shown in the following chart:

Gut Bacteria	Hormone Connection
Estrabolome	The gut bacteria responsible for metabolizing estrogen and preventing estrogen from recirculating in the bloodstream
Thyroid and the microbiome	Converting T4 into T3, the more biologically active form of the thyroid hormone, and absorbing selenium and zinc from food—all gut bacteria activity
Progesterone and the microbiome	Part of the microbiome includes *Candida*, a form of yeast that overgrows in conditions of low progesterone
Insulin and the microbiome	Gut bacteria balances blood sugar, keeping insulin levels balanced as well

According to the National Institutes of Health, "A person's core microbiome is formed in the first years of life but can change over time in response to different factors including diet, medications, and environmental exposures." This mutability is good to know about, because those who eat a healthy diet tend to have a gut microbiome that continually transforms as they get older—a hallmark of healthy aging. For those whose diet is less than optimal, there is less overall microbial diversity, triggering more inflammation, hormone imbalances, and accelerated aging.

Your microbiome also affects the *circulation* of your hormones. Some of the bacteria are responsible for re-circulating the estrogen in your system, while others are responsible for eating up "dirty" estrogen, or the toxic estrogen metabolites that make us sick. The term "dirty estrogen" refers to escalating levels of estrone, a by-product of the estrogen in our bodies, along with xenoestrogens (synthetic or natural compounds imitating estrogen) from the environment. Gut bacteria are responsible for ridding the body of these metabolites. This process prevents conditions and patterns we have discussed, such as estrogen dominance, insulin resistance, PCOS, endometriosis, thyroid disorders, and infertility.

I think of the microbiome as an enormous factory, teeming with activity. The hormones enter your gut, your microbiome gets activated, chopping them up (well, not literally!) and sending them off to the right places in your body, and your organs do what they need to do in receiving the hormones and making sure everything works as it should. Everybody's happy.

But if your gut isn't working well, for whatever reason—say, a high intake of processed food, food dyes, food additives, medications, and/or overexposure to environmental toxins—then your microbiome shifts gears in a negative way. This is called *dysbiosis*. Toxic metabolites and hormones build up, triggering the leaky gut, inflammation, and hormone imbalances. If not stopped, this process can lead to full expression of disease.

This relationship between hormones and the gut is mutually beneficial, by the way. It's not just your gut that needs to work for your hormones; your hormones also influence the health of your gut. It's a constant back-and-forth. So, when women lose progesterone for whatever reason, or they retain estrogen, or they go through menopause, we see shifts in the microbiome itself, causing all sorts of digestive issues. This is the *why* of when pregnant women get reflux, perimenopausal women suffer bloating, or menopausal women are constipated. Progesterone drops, for example, can lead to more *Candida*, or yeast overgrowth; estrogen drops can lead to poor gut motility or to constipation.

Here's another extremely important thing to know: A balanced gut microbiome means less systemic inflammation. Dysbiosis can lead to many health problems, including obesity, Type 2 diabetes, inflammatory bowel disease, celiac disease, liver disease, cancers of the colon and liver, and neurologic conditions such as Alzheimer's and Parkinson's diseases.

Fat Malabsorption—The New Epidemic?

I'm finding over and over again that everyone, from babies and toddlers to adults, is spilling a ton of fat in their stool. And this issue, which I unfortunately keep encountering, is linked to behavioral issues, sensory issues, hormone disruption, and autoimmune disease—and that's just a starting list. Here's what happens when you spill fat.

First, fat is needed to make cholesterol, the building block of hormones. So, when you're losing fat, you're already behind the eight ball when it comes to hormonal balance. You can't stabilize insulin or blood sugar because you need a certain amount of fat to do so. Those levels hop all over the place, and before you know it, you're insulin resistant. This is one of the reasons women with weight issues tend to have hormone issues. Even if you are overweight you can still spill fat, and if you are very thin, you can spill the meager amount of fat you're eating as well.

When I explain this situation to my underweight patients who are striving for an abnormal idea of super-thinness, they're *shocked*. They protest that they don't have a weight issue when actually they do. It's quite unfortunate that in this country have a "weight issue" means being overweight. And being underweight wreaks havoc on all the hormones, too. If your BMI (body mass index) or body fat percentage drops below 19 or 20 percent, you're going to have a really rough time in perimenopause and menopause, as you won't have the buffer of body fat to weather the hormone fluctuations.

Fat is needed for brain development and cognitive function. I often wonder if the growing prevalence of neuro-cognitive and neuro-inflammatory disorders—including sensory-processing disorder, ADHD, anxiety, depression, and global brain fog—can be linked to low cholesterol levels in the blood secondary to fat malabsorption, which in turn leads to low levels of hormones, which then affects brain power.

Further, the microbiome itself can't be stable because there's an increased histamine response in response to fat loss. This response can lead to chronic food intolerances, food allergies, and immune responses. Fortunately, stool samples can pick up fat malabsorption and help guide recommendations for treatment.

This histamine response happened recently to my daughter. She had an allergic reaction to a bee sting, and six months later she can't tolerate shrimp anymore—her gut isn't healthy, because her body's response to the bee sting changed her microbiome. When we get her gut back on track, her allergic reactions should decrease.

Healthy Fats Are Your Gut's BFF

Did you know that the building block of the body's hormones is the fatty substance known as cholesterol? That's right, the very substance you hear scary things about actually helps make your hormones.

There are two types of cholesterol, HDL and LDL, along with triglycerides. HDL (high-density lipoprotein) is considered the "good" cholesterol because healthy levels may protect against heart attack and stroke. HDL is also responsible for carrying LDL (low-density lipoprotein) cholesterol away from the arteries and back to the liver, where the LDL is broken down so it can be excreted. LDL cholesterol is considered the "bad" cholesterol since it can clog your arteries and lead to heart disease or strokes.

Cholesterol has become one of those scary words in the health news, because too much LDL cholesterol can lead to heart disease. But lowering cholesterol levels below 130 mg/dL leads to hormone depletion. Without proper levels of cholesterol, you can't build your hormones or your neurotransmitters, which keep your brain and body healthy.

Like many areas of health and nutrition, it's not all or nothing; it's the sweet spot we should be aiming for. Women who have a low body weight or low body-fat percentage often have low levels of female hormones (estrogen and progesterone) that, in turn, impact fertility, menstrual cycles, blood sugar levels, and overall energy.

How Your Pancreas and Gallbladder Affect Your Hormones

News alert: Your pancreas and gallbladder are part of your overall digestive system. These organs are thought of separately in Western medicine, but they are considered an important united part of gut health in Eastern medicine. And yes, they affect your hormone levels, too, by influencing the metabolism of dietary fat and the regulation of blood sugar.

About Your Pancreas

The pancreas is an incredibly important organ but one that most people don't think a lot about unless they are diabetic or have developed cancer. Located in the middle section of the belly, slightly under the rib cage, the pancreas has several functions.

First, it secretes digestive enzymes involved in the digestive process, allowing the breakdown of the foods we've eaten. This is fundamental to the digestion of fats, protein, and carbohydrates. Pancreatic injury can result in fat malabsorption.

Also, the pancreas is responsible for the production and regulation of the hormone insulin, which is what manages the amount of sugar, or glucose, in the blood. Type 1 diabetes is a genetic disease in which insulin is not made; those with Type 1 must regulate the levels on their own, with regular injections of insulin. This is pancreatic malfunctioning at its worst. Type 2 diabetes is not genetic and is more common, caused when the body makes insulin but can't use it properly. This is often the result of an unhealthy gut microbiome, leaky gut, or fat malabsorption, which is what happens when the body is not able to digest fats effectively.

The pancreas, along with the digestive process, determines the body's insulin levels. Insulin, in turn, influences so many functions of the body: weight, inflammation level, and levels of estrogen, thyroid hormones, and androgen as well.

About Your Gallbladder

The gallbladder is a very small, pear-shaped organ nestled under the liver. It is responsible for the storage and release of a liquid called *bile*, which is made in the liver, every time you eat. The bile moves into ducts and then breaks down fats into a substance called *chyme* so the body can then digest it properly in the small intestine. This organ is critical for fat digestion and delivery.

The Hormone Response to Sluggish Pancreas and Gallbladder

The gallbladder and pancreas work in tandem. First, bile is released to break down fats into chyme, and the pancreas assists by providing the right enzymes to package the chyme and deliver it to where it needs to go. But if these two organs become sluggish or overburdened owing to poor diet, stress, lack of sleep, and/or environmental toxins, the process can't happen. Fat malabsorption results instead, or fat spills into your stool rather than getting packaged and helping to build hormones. This in turn creates low *qi*, as they would say in Chinese medicine, or kidney and gallbladder meridian deficiency, as in Ayurveda. And true to East-West medicine, lab results for patients with this condition show high amounts of fat in their stool cultures.

Oh, That Dreaded Bloat

Bloating is one of the most common complaints I hear. My patients tell me, "OMG, I woke up and I look pregnant! I didn't do anything. I can't even fit into my favorite jeans!" I know the feeling, as I've had periods of bad bloating and had to make some changes in my diet.

Bloat can make you feel fat and uncomfortable, but it's not the same as weight gain. There are several reasons for bloating to occur:

- You're not getting enough dietary fiber. You need at least 40 grams of fiber each day, which is a lot more than you'd think. A cup of lentils or black beans is 15 grams, and who eats three or four cups of beans during the day? Not me! A cup of Brussels sprouts is only 4 grams, as much as a baked potato. Without enough fiber, your gut cannot move food through the process known as peristalsis, and you can retain more water.
- You're eating too many foods that are hard to digest, like red meats, raw fruits and veggies, sugar, greasy or fried foods, and processed fast food.
- Your production of digestive enzymes is decreasing, which is a normal part of the aging process. Taking a supplement with your meal should help tremendously.
- You have leaky gut, leading to malabsorption of nutrients.
- You have dysbiosis or microbial imbalance, triggering *Candida* overgrowth.
- You have fibroids or undiagnosed ovarian issues. Be sure to ask for a vaginal ultrasound for a thorough ovarian evaluation at every checkup to make sure there's no physical cause of bloating.
- You have hormonal bloating. This, of course, is the biggest thing that often gets missed. Higher estrogen levels cause bloating, since estrogen influences water retention, and too much estrogen can slow down how fast your gut can process nutrients.

Balancing your hormones and your digestive system is key to de-bloating. In the meantime, one old-fashioned treatment that is comforting and bloat reducing is to rub a thick layer of castor oil on your abdomen, cover with a piece of cotton flannel, and then put a heating pad on top. Lie down and let the heat permeate your abdomen for at least thirty minutes.

Supplements for Gut–Hormone Health

There are several supplements I recommend that support gut health, especially if you have a history of digestive issues, bloating, and hormonal imbalance. You can find more details about choosing the best supplements in Chapter 9.

Digestive Enzymes

Digestive enzymes are an amazingly useful supplement I give to nearly all my patients. A top-quality supplement will work beautifully, especially for those who need just a little bit of support—one pill a day, usually with your heaviest meal, either lunch or dinner. Those with more serious digestive issues need to take one pill with every meal.

The reason for taking digestive enzymes? The digestive enzymes are proteins that stimulate digestion. There are three types produced by the pancreas: proteases (to digest proteins), lipases (to break down fats), and amylases (to break down carbohydrates into simple sugars). If fat malabsorption is the problem, look for a supplement with ox bile and lipase to break down fats effectively.

Probiotics

The World Health Organization describes probiotics as "live microorganisms which when administered in adequate amounts confer a health benefit to the host." In other words, a probiotic is a microbe that is therapeutic in some way. A probiotic supplement has one or more strains of the beneficial bacteria that live in your gut, and it can help regulate digestion and improve your gut microbiome.

I am a big proponent of probiotics, but there's a lot of debate about their effectiveness. Some claim that you can't fundamentally change the microbiome, that it is genetically hardwired in some way. In addition, there is a lot of variability in probiotic quality; supplements are *not* regulated by the U.S. Food and Drug Administration, so consumers are dependent on the brand or company doing their own due diligence, verifying quality through various certifications, including the GMP (Good Manufacturing Products) seal and an NSF International or USP (US Pharmacopeia) seal.

It's best to get the majority of your probiotics from food, as each food has a unique microbiome of its own. Supplementation is helpful since most of us don't vary our foods and our food quality can be an issue. Processed and packaged foods, for example, don't have a rich microbial footprint to help the gut in comparison to fresh foods prepared at home and varied seasonally. When shopping for a probiotic supplement, look for encapsulated probiotics with a proven track record of viability. The pill should have at least 50 billion CFU (colony-forming units), with clear labeling of the strains of bacteria and their amounts. Take one pill each morning with your breakfast. I often recommend rotating your probiotics every few months to maintain microbiome diversity.

Prebiotics

A prebiotic is the food the probiotics use to do their work. Prebiotics are derived from plant fibers and are found in many different fruits, vegetables, and whole grains. Some of my favorite prebiotic foods are chicory root, artichoke leaves, and dandelion greens.

Some patients can't tolerate probiotics, as they already have bacterial overgrowth, but they do better with prebiotics that balance the microbiome indirectly. Inulin, for example, is a commonly used prebiotic supplement.

Glutamine

This is one of my all-time favorite supplements for good gut health. Glutamine is an amino acid that helps protect the lining of the gastro-intestinal tract (the mucosa), healing and sealing a leaky gut. Many of our patients at CentreSpringMD have had incredible success with glutamine in just a few weeks. I recommend taking it in powder form, as it's easier to absorb. Start with 500 milligrams and work up to 1 to 2 grams after two weeks.

Aloe Vera Juice

The juice of the succulent plant aloe vera is known to help balance the gut bacteria and improve the gut lining. You need to drink only 1 to 2 ounces (2 to 4 tablespoons) every day. Be sure to get only pure juice, as many aloe vera drinks are high in sugar.

Gut Health = Bone Health

Gut health is linked to both osteopenia and osteoporosis. As hormone levels fall in premature menopause, perimenopause, and menopause, bone health starts to decline. Hormones are needed to build healthy bones, but when we apply the integrative or functional approach to bone health, the gut becomes ground zero.

The gut, after all, determines how we absorb the nutrients needed to build healthy bones, and how much inflammation our bodies are carrying. These factors become even more important in the face of declining hormone levels. Producing less estrogen means there's less bone deposition, so there is a tendency to have frailer and thinner bones.

Develop Your Gut Smarts

Yes, you have graduated from Hormone University and have also begun to acquire gut smarts, which may be even more important to your health. If you are not sure where to begin in your quest for hormone power, know that it really does start with the gut. And when the gut is thriving, you really can trust your gut to deliver good health.

In my Thirty-Day Hormone Reset (which is presented in Chapter 9), step 1 is all about getting gut healthy again. But first, take a few moments to digest (sorry, had to!) the information presented in this chapter and evaluate your own gut health at this point.

chapter 7

Hormones and Nutrition

If your gut is ground zero for hormone health, then your nutrition is a close second. Would you run a car without any gas in the tank? I am pretty sure the answer is no. Then why run your body without fuel? It happens every day.

Hormone balance is a symphony whose performance depends on the instruments in the happy orchestra of the body to be playing their respective parts. The gut needs to do its gut stuff, but even when it's switched on and ready, without the right food to provide nutrients, it can't work to balance the body's hormones.

In practice, I see firsthand how a lack of essential nutrients—including the B vitamins, iron, vitamin D, omega-3 and omega-9 fats, selenium, zinc—okay, I'll stop! All these nutrients impact hormone health. How? It's simple. Every hormone pathway in the body is dependent on receiving key nutrients. And if your diet is unable to provide these nutrients, back to Hormone Hell, you go.

The Hormone Pathway

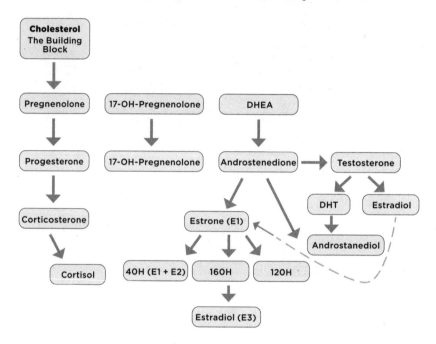

The Top Ten Nutrients You Need

Vitamins and Minerals

B Vitamins

The B vitamins are key micronutrients involved in regulating hormone pathways and neurotransmitters. More specifically, the B vitamins are involved in metabolizing estrogen, balancing thyroid function, and supporting cortisol and progesterone production. They are all critical pieces of the hormone puzzle. But let's look at what are essential B vitamins:

- B_1 (thiamine)—activates the detoxification pathways in the liver, specifically phase 1, allowing hormone metabolites to get broken down.
- B_2 (riboflavin)—supports detoxification, energy production, fatty acid profiles, and the thyroid.
- B_3 (niacin)—regulates cholesterol, the building block of hormones, as well as growth hormone production and estrogen metabolism.
- B_5 (pantothenic acid)—supports estrogen and progesterone production, improves fatigue, relieves headaches.
- B_6 (pyridoxal 5' phosphate [P5P])—supports liver function; it also binds to estrogen, progesterone, and testosterone, helping to bind and break down excess levels of these hormones. This vitamin actually lowers the risk for hormone-related cancers.
- B_7 (biotin)—improves ovulation and egg production; works to strengthen and thicken hair and nails.
- B_9 (folate)—breaks down homocysteine levels, an inflammation marker, while lowering ACTH, the hormone that leads to high blood pressure; also reduces the risk for birth defects and protects against anemia.
- B_{12} (cobalamin)—works to improve energy, detoxification, melatonin production, and memory.

About Methylation

Ideally, the B vitamin supplements you take are methylated, meaning they have an additional carbon group that allows for more easy absorption.

Methylation is a physiological pathway that you need to know about if you have the MTHFR (methylenetetrahydrofolate reductase) genetic mutation, which can impair certain chemical processes in the body. The primary function of the MTHFR enzyme is to help the body produce folate (the B vitamin), which you need to create DNA, to detoxify, and to balance hormones and neurotransmitters. If the MTHFR gene mutates, a range of health conditions can result.

This is a common mutation, now found in 30 to 40 percent of the population. If you have the MTHFR mutation, it is hard to absorb and efficiently use nutrients, hormones, and different other substances. This can lead to a B vitamin deficiency within the cells, causing hormone disruption, mood and focus issues, and increased toxic load. The easiest way to manage this situation is with supplements that are methylated.

Methylation adds methyl groups to supplements so that the body can better absorb those supplements. I recommend that everyone test for this mutation, either with a simple blood or a saliva test. Or, you could take methylated supplements, which don't cause harm. I'm not sure why this mutation is becoming more prevalent; it may be due to overall increased environmental toxicity, which encourages mutations and cellular changes.

Vitamin D

It is common to have a vitamin D deficiency. Without proper levels of vitamin D in the body, there are many hormone-mediated symptoms. For instance, low vitamin D levels have been linked to the following:

- Low estrogen levels
- Lower levels of androgens
- Insulin resistance
- Osteopenia and osteoporosis
- Poor immune function

We need sunlight to trigger the metabolism of vitamin D in the skin, so if you always use a sunscreen or have darker skin tone, your production of vitamin D can be affected. Also, vitamin D is a fat-soluble vitamin; compromised gut health and issues with fat malabsorption can cause a chronic vitamin D deficiency, even with supplementation.

Iron

Iron is needed for optimal thyroid function and for healthy red blood cells. Low levels of red blood cells cause anemia. Fibroids, heavy menstrual flow, and low iron intake in vegan and vegetarian diets are frequent reasons I find anemia or low ferritin (the iron storage protein) among the women who come to my practice. Low iron levels can trigger the following:

- Breathlessness
- Fatigue
- High cortisol/adrenal fatigue
- Insulin resistance
- Low blood pressure
- Low progesterone levels
- Poor thyroid function

Adding iron-rich foods to your diet or supplementing with iron is often necessary if you are experiencing any of these symptoms.

Magnesium

Magnesium, the "miracle micronutrient" as I call it, is a co-factor for hormones and neurotransmitters. It's involved in hundreds of pathways in the body, and deficiencies of magnesium are often at the root of many hormone-based symptoms. Low magnesium levels have been linked to the following:

- Diabetes
- High estrogen levels
- IBS
- Insulin resistance
- Insomnia
- Low progesterone levels
- PMS
- Poor thyroid function
- Thyroid disorders

There are many different forms of magnesium, but a blended chelated form tackles most of the conditions on this list. A chelated magnesium is one in which multiple forms of magnesium are blended together; for example, it may be a compound of magnesium threonate, glycinate, and citrate.

Selenium

A must for the thyroid gland, selenium is needed to convert T4 into the more metabolically active T3. This powerful mineral is directly involved in the production of the thyroid hormones. It helps prevent oxidative damage to the thyroid and strengthens the immune system.

Vitamin E

A fat-soluble vitamin, vitamin E is known to encourage healthy skin and hair, and it also improves hormone function. Vitamin E can aid the body in the following ways:

- Improve cholesterol profiles, boosting HDL levels
- Improve insulin resistance
- Increase progesterone levels
- Lower LDL cholesterol levels
- Lower testosterone levels

Given that vitamin E is fat-soluble, many of my patients with fat malabsorption suffer from a vitamin E deficiency.

Zinc

Zinc is an important micronutrient for hormone balance, immune function, and metabolism. Zinc is also a co-factor in testosterone production, helps boost production of the growth hormone, and supports cortisol production. Low zinc levels can cause the following:

- High cortisol
- High estrogen
- Infertility
- Low libido
- Low progesterone
- PMS

Deficiencies of zinc can be caused by hormone replacement therapy or birth control, medications, or low dietary intake.

The Healthy Fats

Omega-3 Fats

Nourishing for the brain and containing the cholesterol the body needs for hormone production, omega-3 fats also help reduce inflammation in the body and relieve symptoms of anxiety and depression. Low omega-3 levels are linked to the following:

- High androgens
- Infertility
- Inflammation
- Insulin resistance
- Low estrogen levels
- Low progesterone levels
- Low testosterone levels

Increasing your intake of omega-3 fats has been found to be helpful for overall hormone support.

Omega-9 Fats

Omega-9 fats can be produced in your body and are found naturally in some foods, like avocados, olive oil, and almonds. They can reduce inflammation and allow for better insulin sensitivity. Omega-9 fats are also involved in estrogen metabolism, improving the breakdown and detoxification of estrogen.

Probiotics

Probiotics were discussed in Chapter 6, but getting the right balance of good bacteria in the gut is why probiotics make my Top Ten nutrient list. Probiotics have been linked to hormone balance in a number of ways, as follows:

- Balanced cortisol levels
- Improved estrogen metabolism
- Improved insulin resistance
- Improved progesterone balance
- Lower *Candida*
- Lower androgens
- Lower LDL cholesterol levels

The research concerning probiotics is fascinating, with specific microbial strains tied to specific conditions; for example, an overgrowth of the *Clostridia* bacteria is tied to PCOS, while other bacteria, collectively known as the *estrabolome*, are needed to help improve uptake of estrogen and prevent recirculation of estrogen into the bloodstream.

Hormone-Friendly Foods

Where should most of the nutrients your body needs come from? From our food. Food is our first medicine, and without it or if we neglect it, hormone balance and vitality continue to be a distant goal. It should not be hard to meet our food goals, to successfully nourish ourselves and our families, or even to find the eating plan that works for you. But it is.

What has happened instead is that food in some ways is seen as our enemy. That's because there are good foods and bad foods, there's too much food, there's fashion in foods, and overall general confusion about food. It's something my patients complain about every day.

It does not have to be this way. Getting the nutrients your hormones need can happen naturally—as long as your gut is working properly—when you stick to whole, minimally processed foods. I know your eyes are rolling right now because you have heard this several times before, and you know it is easier said than done. Every Superwoman I meet either is too busy to get in the kitchen, is afraid of the kitchen, or is so stressed that meal planning is the last thing on her to-do list.

In my Thirty-Day Hormone Reset (Chapter 9), I advise you on how to get back into the kitchen, how to love and see food as your superpower, and how to ditch unhealthy habits for good ones. But before you go there, let's discuss the hormone traps that are in your way.

Five Hormone Traps

Hormone Trap #1: Inflammatory Foods

It's rampant everywhere. Inflammation: your body on fire. And where does this inflammation come from? Nearly 75 to 80 percent of the time you get it from your gut.

Inflammation directly impacts your hormones, altering insulin levels, increasing androgen levels, and depleting nutrients. It is always my first goal when working with patients to get their inflammation down.

The Top Inflammatory Foods—Major Offenders

Here are the major offenders—the foods that most often cause inflammation and that wear down gut function. I bet some of these will look familiar.

Alcohol

Alcohol has been found guilty of spiking insulin levels, causing yeast overgrowth, worsening estrogen dominance, and lowering testosterone. Ideally, any alcohol consumed should be in limited amounts—under four drinks per week.

Artificial Sweeteners

A microbiome disruptor, artificial sweeteners like aspartame and sucralose trigger insulin resistance and estrogen dominance. Early research suggests it contributes to thyroid dysfunction as well.

Chemicals and Food Additives

Preservatives, food dyes, binders, and fillers all affect hormone health by disrupting the microbiome, causing high cortisol levels and insulin resistance. Many of these chemicals and food additives are endocrine disrupters, and they impact estrogen levels, increasing the risk of hormone-based cancers (including breast cancer). These preservatives include the following:

- BHT
- BPA
- DHT
- Food dyes
- Parabens
- PFOA

Dairy Products

An intolerance or allergy to casein, the protein in dairy, or to lactose, the sugar found in dairy, impacts digestive health, worsening insulin resistance, *Candida* overgrowth, and altered estrogen and progesterone levels, since most dairy products contain hormones.

Gluten

Gluten is the protein found in wheat and some other grains. Gluten intolerance and celiac disease can cause an immune reaction in the gut, creating leaky gut, high cortisol, poor thyroid function, low progesterone, and estrogen dominance.

Meats

Excessive consumption of meat in any form slows down the digestion, increases insulin resistance, and can impact estrogen levels in both men and women. Factory-farmed meat, which often has added hormones, further impacts the body's hormone profile, raising estrogen levels and worsening estrogen dominance.

Saturated Fats and Trans Fats

Found in meats, dairy products, and packaged and processed foods, saturated fats and trans fats impact blood sugar levels, the gut, and estrogen metabolism (higher estrogen levels). In recent studies, trans fats, which are hydrogenated vegetable oils, have been found to lower testosterone levels in men and women, while high levels of saturated fats impact the gut microbiome and cholesterol levels, contributing to insulin resistance and estrogen dominance.

Soy Products

With the abundance of products made from soybeans used as a substitute for meat protein, I have to include it on this list of offenders. Although soy products promote estrogen production through their isoflavones, too much soy, especially highly processed soy, can impact fertility, trigger early puberty, and interfere with production of the thyroid hormones. Highly processed soy has a negative impact on hormones, while fermented soy actually can benefit estrogen metabolism due to the isoflavones.

Sugars

A direct disruptor of insulin, sugar triggers the highs and lows that make us insulin resistant. It also spikes the androgen, estrogen, and testosterone levels. And, yes, this is true of all sugars. For those with insulin sensitivity, even the natural sugars found in fruits can be an issue.

Snacks—Simple and Refined Carbohydrates

They are yummy and easy to grab, but snacks are not helping your hormones. The entire family of simple and refined carbohydrates (chips, cookies, and so on) can trigger insulin resistance, high cortisol levels, and sluggish thyroid function.

If you find that you have systemic inflammation, eliminating these pro-inflammatory foods is critical. This step is likely not forever, but it is necessary for a period of time to get the inflammation down and your gut back on track. The topic of inflammation is covered later, in connection with the Thirty-Day Hormone Reset (Chapter 9).

Refined Carbohydrates, Sugar, and Your Hormones

As we get older, we become less tolerant of sugar in all its forms, from simple carbohydrates like table sugar, baked goods, white bread, and pasta, all the way to white rice and packaged foods. Sugar spikes the insulin, which makes the blood sugar levels go haywire and then triggers fat storage. The ups and downs of sugar and insulin levels—well, that's Hormone Hell.

Sugar is a drug and should be labeled that way. Our taste buds change as we consume more sugar, making us crave even more sugar. It's addictive. We use sugar in our foods because it tastes good, and when we're having a bad day, something sweet can make us feel better in the moment. We also use sugar as an instant pick-me-up when we're tired, but then we crash quickly, leaving us wanting more sugar. And the cycle continues.

In America, we have a culture of over-sweetening practically everything, so our taste buds have adapted to this higher sugar load. The easy availability and low cost of sugar is a fairly recent development in the long span of human history, as sugar used to be a luxury item. Our bodies aren't designed to process a lot of sugar, which is why it should be used in limited amounts.

Many consumers are unaware of the added sugars in the foods they buy. Sugar is snuck in by manufacturers who know it will make their items taste "better" and leave you wanting more. Why, for example, is there sugar in ketchup, when tomatoes are naturally sweet? One patient told me she bought some seasoned salt without looking at the label—really, who would?—and when she happened to glance at it, she was shocked that the second ingredient was sugar. In a salt mixture!

The best advice here is to always read the label of any packaged or prepared foods you buy. It's a habit that will not only save you money but also improve your eating habits. The fat, sugar, protein, fiber, calories, and any fortifications included must be listed, so if you know what your daily requirements are, you can judge accordingly. In regard to this, one of the easiest mistakes to make is to overlook the serving size. If you're in a hurry and don't look carefully, it's easy to miss that the nutrition facts are based on a small serving size—smaller than you would consider.

A less recognized problem in sugar management occurs when sugar is in liquid form. When I posted a YouTube video about some food myths, I mentioned that some ready-made blended smoothies contain a whopping 40 to 50 grams of sugar. This is why fruit-juice-based smoothies are best avoided, thereby avoiding the sugar load and resulting insulin spikes.

Yes, green smoothies that are veggie-based are good for you, but if you're going to be drinking all your meals or snacks, you need to ensure that the drink is balanced with protein and fiber. It's far better to eat half a grapefruit than to have a glass of grapefruit juice. The fruit has much more fiber, takes longer to eat, and won't cause the insulin spike that juice does.

Be aware also that alcohol is processed in the body as sugar. If you avoid sugar all day long, but then have two glasses of wine every night, that's a lot of sugar to process.

Sugar substitutes are not a solution. Drinking diet soda and eating sugar-free candies or baked goods will still cause an insulin spike, because your body perceives the fake sugar as real sugar and the microbiome is disrupted, leading to higher estrogen and insulin levels, and landing you in Hormone Hell.

Fortunately, you can retrain your sweet tooth. You honestly will lose your taste for added sugar when you start to cut down, and you won't really need a lot to get the desired sweetness. Lowering your sugar consumption to the point where you really don't want it is a prime hormone goal. And you will eventually be able to satisfy any sugar cravings with a small serving of fruit, which contains natural sugars and fiber, having less effect on your insulin and blood sugar levels.

Your hormone goal: total sugar under 25 grams per day, or 3 to 4 teaspoons at most.

Look Out for Hidden Sugars

A sugar by any other name is still as sweet! Any of the following items are still processed in your body as sugar: agave syrup, barley malt, corn sweetener, dextrose, fructose, fruit juice concentrate, galactose, glucose,

golden syrup, high fructose corn syrup, honey, lactose, malt syrup, malt-
ose, molasses, monk fruit, pure cane sugar, raw sugar, rice syrup, stevia,
sucrose, treacle.

Hormone Trap #2: Caffeine

When I was growing up, there were no coffee shops like Starbucks on
every corner. The easy availability of take-out coffee drinks today has
made us all over-caffeinated. Add energy drinks and some sodas to this
and your caffeine load gets supersized.

Here's what caffeine does to your hormones: It exaggerates the
production of stress hormones, specifically cortisol, and it can increase
your estrogen levels. Studies have shown that, in women, increased caffeine intake is associated with decreased testosterone.

So, caffeine does impact your hormones—but there is a sweet spot.
A clean, organic coffee can actually boost cardiovascular health, clear
brain fog, and add energy—as long as its consumption is kept under
4 to 6 ounces (½ to ¾ cup) per day.

If you switch to decaffeinated coffee, you still want to stay between
4 and 6 ounces (½ to ¾ cup), as the decaffeinating process can actually
create a more "toxic" coffee, higher in a chemical called methylene
chloride, unless it is labeled as decaffeinated through a Swiss water
process, which uses only water to remove the caffeine.

Hormone Trap #3: Gluten-Free and Dairy-Free

Gluten is a protein found in wheat, barley, and rye. If you have a sensitivity or allergy to it, or if you have celiac disease, which is the genetic

inability to process gluten, consumption of gluten foods can lead to inflammation, which as we discussed can be responsible for damage to the villi in your intestine, intensifying the problems of a leaky gut. Dairy products contain hormones, and as mentioned, the protein and sugar in these foods can be problematic for many with an already leaky gut or *Candida* overgrowth.

But once you remove the dairy and gluten from your diet, you can fall into another hormone trap—foods high in simple carbohydrates and/or sugar, added to improve taste. That is, going gluten-free and dairy-free means continuing to mindfully practice choosing real, un-processed foods and saving the substitutes for the occasional treat.

Hormone Trap #4: Fasting

There has been much written and debated about the role of fasting for overall health, and intermittent fasting is particularly recommended for weight loss. But what impact does fasting have on the body's hor-mones and hormone balance?

Fasting has been a mainstay for many cultures and traditions over time. Every major religion has some element of fasting as a part of its rituals and practices. This is not an accident. There are many benefits to fasting, regardless of the interval between eating times (eight hours, twelve hours, twenty-four hours, etc.).

Our general understanding of fasting has shown that it accom-plishes the following:

Improves blood sugar balance and insulin resistance. The mechanism of action here is overall gut rest and lowered caloric intake. Gut rest is a central Eastern concept as well; both Chinese and Ayurvedic medi-cine stress the importance of resting the gut for optimal digestive and metabolic health. While the recommendations vary based on the patient, a twelve-hour gut rest is considered ideal, with clear three- to four-hour intervals between eating times throughout the day, allowing for adequate digestion. This fasting interval is included in the Thirty-Day Hormone Reset (Chapter 9).

Improves blood pressure and lowers triglycerides and bad cholesterol. The mechanism of action regarding blood pressure and triglycerides is similar to that for blood sugar: gut rest and lowered caloric intake spark *autophagy*, or the orderly cleansing or rebooting of cells after a period of rest and deprivation. It's kind of like cleaning out your closet; once you get rid of the clutter, you can think and see more clearly. Thus, with autophagy, fasting stimulates a detox and removal of old cells, dead cells, or particles we don't need, resetting our cellular health.

Reduces inflammation. Fasting has been shown to give an overall reduction of inflammatory symptoms, including joint pain, rashes, brain fog, and risks for diseases of inflammation, including heart disease, cancer, and autoimmune diseases.

Weight loss. Short-term fasting (or intermittent fasting) for twelve to fifteen hours per day—and yes, here's the catch—has been shown to help with weight loss as long as it is limited to a few months. But when fasting continues past this time, there is a gradual reduction in metabolic rate, which can actually lead to weight gain and hormone disruption.

And then, in regard to fasting, there is the debate about women and their hormones. I am not sure you are going to welcome my stance on this, but let's approach fasting with an EastWest perspective. That means, as with all things, there is a sweet spot.

Short-term or intermittent fasting does indeed jump-start your metabolism, reduce caloric intake, improve insulin resistance, and increase levels of growth hormone, which is the anti-aging hormone that regulates muscle mass, testosterone levels, and sleep quality. But when it's done for an extended time—greater than three months, or continuously without any breaks—this type of fasting could cause a decrease in estrogen and progesterone production. There is also early research showing that this prolonged fasting disrupts the thyroid/adrenal axis, creating a state of adrenal fatigue and high cortisol, depleting the thyroid function and worsening this hormone imbalance.

So, where's the sweet spot? It's in cycling through intermittent fasting—maybe a five-day-on/two-day-off approach, or fasting one or two days per week to reset metabolism and stimulate autophagy. That is what works for most women, but if you are highly stressed, not sleeping, or already dealing with fluctuations or depletion in estrogen, progesterone, or thyroid levels, fasting should be no longer than twelve hours and definitely not a starting point for achieving hormone balance.

Hormone Trap #5: Keto

Another trending fad, the keto diet is one so many of my patients ask me about, and some have even had some success with losing weight, clearing up brain fog, and breaking their long-standing sugar addiction. The keto diet does help us with Hormone Traps 1, 2, and 3, as it removes refined carbohydrates and sugars, and it increases healthy fats, which as we know are the building blocks of hormones.

A true keto diet is defined as one that is high in fat and low in carbohydrates and sugars, allowing the body to break fat down into ketones as a source of energy. Fish, avocados, poultry, meats, eggs, and low-carb veggies are examples of foods "allowed" on the keto diet.

These are all foods that help combat insulin resistance and reduce inflammation.

But the keto diet can raise cholesterol levels, including LDL (bad) cholesterol, increasing concerns for those with known cardiovascular disease. Many keto eating plans allow up to 75 grams of fat, including saturated fats, to help the body get to "ketosis," or the fat-burning stage. The carbohydrate load can be extremely low, often as low as 25 grams, causing mood swings, trouble sleeping, and more hormone disruption.

All this added fat can increase estrogen levels, worsening estrogen dominance, or the storage of estrogen throughout the body. Estrogen dominance, in turn, makes insulin resistance worse, and together this pattern wears down the thyroid function.

Here we are again, trying to find the sweet spot, embracing the idea that fat is good and needed, but knowing that too much of it comes with a risk to hormones and other health markers. In the Thirty-Day Hormone Reset (Chapter 9), we moderate many of these ideas in a way that works for hormone balance, good energy levels, mood, and overall health and vitality.

Superfoods for Hormone Health

The foods on the following list are all good for your gut, which means they will improve the production and detoxification of your hormones. They are high in fiber, high in protein, are healthy fats, and/or are high in antioxidants; for that reason, there is some overlap in the categories listed. The nutrient goal here is to include these foods in your daily diet, or, when the opportunity presents itself, pick these foods over other choices.

High-Fiber Foods

Fiber is essential for hormone balance because it is involved in the breakdown of estrogen and the management of blood sugar and insulin resistance. Fiber also supports gut motility and keeps us feeling full and satiated.

Fiber comes in two forms: soluble and insoluble. *Soluble fiber* is digestive; that is, it dissolves in water and forms a gel-like substance to slow digestion. *Insoluble fiber* can't dissolve in fluids, and so it helps speed up digestion. It allows foods to form a softer and bulkier stool for more regular elimination.

The goal is to get a minimum of 40 grams of total fiber daily, so as to support hormone production and detoxification. The highest levels of fiber are found in chia seeds and oats.

Food	Grams of Fiber
Almonds, 1 ounce	3.5
Apples, 1 medium, with skin	4.5
Artichokes, 1 medium	6.2
Avocados, 1 cup	10.0
Beets (cooked), 1 cup	3.8
Broccoli (cooked), 1 cup	5.0
Carrots (cooked), 1 medium	1.5
Chia seeds, 1 ounce	10.0
Chickpeas (cooked), 1 cup	12.5
Guava, 1 cup	9.0
Kidney beans (cooked), 1 cup	12.2
Lentils (cooked), 1 cup	15.5

Food	Grams of Fiber
Oats, 1 cup (uncooked)	16.5
Pears, 1 medium, with skin	5.5
Prunes, 10 dried	6.0
Pumpkin, $1/2$ cup, canned	5.0
Raspberries, 1 cup	8.0
Split peas (cooked), 1 cup	16.0

Healthy Fats

Healthy fats are the building blocks for hormones; they also reduce inflammation and support estrogen metabolism. The goal is to get 30 to 40 grams daily.

Food	Type of Fat	Grams of Fat
Almonds, 1 ounce	omega-3 + 9	314.0
Avocado, $1/2$	omega-9 + MCT*	914.7
Chia seeds, 1 ounce	omega-3	38.5
Flax seeds, 1 tablespoon	omega-3	32.95
Macadamia nuts, $1/4$ cup	MCT*	25.2
Olive oil, 1 tablespoon	omega-9	914.0
Salmon, 6 ounces (cooked)	omega-3	318.5
Tuna, 6 ounces (cooked)	omega-3	31.0

*MCT, or medium chain triglycerides, are medium length fatty acids that are used as an energy source in the body. Because they are metabolized differently and convert into ketones, they support metabolic health and digestion.

Clean Protein

Protein as a nutrient preserves muscle mass, keeps blood sugar levels stable, and prevents consumption of refined carbohydrates and sugars. Aim for 3 to 4 ounces of meat-based protein per day, or 8 to 10 ounces of plant-based protein. The goal is to have 80 grams of protein daily.

If you eat meat, try to eat only grass-fed, grass-finished meats if you can afford them. Grass is what grazing animals are meant to eat, but mass-processed animals are fed enormous quantities of grains before slaughter to plump them up. This means you are also consuming whatever antibiotics and other substances have been added to the feed. Grass-fed animals still can be fed grains if they aren't also labeled grass-finished, so always check the label.

Protein Guide
Grams of protein per serving (cooked unless otherwise indicated)
4 ounces = 1/2 cup
8 ounces = 1 cup

Food	Serving Size	Amount
Meats		
Beef		
Ground	4 ounces	28 grams
Steaks	4 ounces	25 grams
Hamburger (large patty)	1	26 grams
Chicken	4 ounces	28–30 grams
Eggs	2 (medium to large)	14–20 grams
Fish	3.5 ounces	25–30 grams
Lamb	3 ounces	21 grams
Turkey, ground	4 ounces	21 grams
Deli meats (turkey, chicken)	2 thick slices	24 grams

Food	Serving Size	Amount
Dairy		
Greek yogurt	8 ounces	22 grams
Cheese		
Parmesan	1 ounce	10 grams
Other	1 ounce	7 grams
Kefir	8 ounces	9 grams
Whole milk	8 ounces	8 grams
Dairy Alternatives		
Almond milk	8 ounces	1 gram
Coconut milk	8 ounces	4 grams
Hemp milk	8 ounces	3 grams
Rice milk	8 ounces	0.7 grams
Soy milk	8 ounces	8 grams
Plant-Based Sources		
Beans (black, navy, pinto, red, kidney, garbanzo)	8 ounces	15 grams
Lentils	8 ounces	18 grams
Soy beans	8 ounces	30 grams
Tempeh	8 ounces	42 grams
Tofu	8 ounces	14 grams
Nuts/Seeds		
Almond butter	1 tablespoon	3.4 grams
Almonds	10	2.5 grams
Cashews	10	5 grams
Peanut butter	1 tablespoon	4 grams
Peanuts	10	5–7 grams
Walnuts	10	12 grams

Food	Serving Size	Amount
Higher-Protein Vegetables		
Artichokes	8 ounces	4–5 grams
Asparagus	8 ounces	4 grams
Brussels sprouts	8 ounces	4 grams
Green peas	8 ounces	8 grams
Kale	8 ounces	3.5 grams
Mushrooms	8 ounces	4 grams
Sweet corn	8 ounces	4 grams

Gut Support

Fermented foods are a part of an EastWest hormone-balancing plan. The process of fermentation improves the food's bacterial diversity, allowing more good bacteria to grow. Here are my favorite fermented foods.

Fermented Foods
  Kefir, preferably made from coconut milk
  Kimchi
  Kombucha
  Miso paste
  Pickles
  Sauerkraut
  Tempeh
  Yogurt with active cultures

For Nutritional Support and Good Fats
  Bone broth
  Coconut oil
  Ghee (clarified butter)

Liver Cleansers

Liver cleansers are foods that support and detoxify the liver, supporting hormone balance, especially estrogen dominance and insulin resistance. Here are a few of my favorites:

Beet greens	Garlic
Broccoli sprouts	Green tea
Cilantro (fresh)	Lemons
Cucumbers	Parsley (fresh)
Dandelion greens	Water
Ginger (fresh)	

Thyroid Support

Nutrients for optimal thyroid function include iron, selenium, magnesium, and iodine, found in these foods:

Almonds	Leafy greens
Brazil nuts	Red meat (grass-fed,
Dark chocolate (no more	grass-finished)
than one square per day!)	Sea vegetables, like nori or
Iodized salt	kelp

Foods to Beat Estrogen Dominance

Estrogen dominance is a hormone pattern common to every phase and cycle of a woman's life. Here are a few foods that help metabolize estrogen, preventing it from being stored in the body:

Broccoli   Kale
Broccoli sprouts   Mushrooms (fresh)
Brussels sprouts   Olive oil
Cauliflower   Salmon
Flax seeds   Turmeric (powder and root)
Fenugreek

Foods to Boost Progesterone

Progesterone levels decline with age, deficiencies in fatty acids, and high stress. Balancing and boosting the progesterone levels saved me in my twenties. These are foods that can help naturally boost your progesterone by providing the phytonutrients needed for *qi* and overall hormone balance:

Avocado   Nuts
Beef   Pumpkin seeds
Chicken   Shrimp
Dark chocolate (1 ounce)   Turkey

Overall Hormone Superstars

If you take a close look at these lists, you'll see that some foods appear a number of times, in different categories—they are true hormone superstars. My short list of hormone-friendly foods includes the following:

Avocado   Dandelion greens
Cruciferous vegetables   Green tea

Leafy greens	Nuts
Fresh-squeezed lemon in water	Olive oil
	Salmon
Meat, organic and grass-fed (chicken, beef, turkey)	Seeds (chia, flax, pumpkin)

With these lists of superfoods, and now that you know the five hormone traps, you may be getting an inkling of what the Thirty-Day Hormone Reset (Chapter 9) will be like. We are almost there.

Common Nutrition Myths

Heard these before? Here are some common myths that we really need to bury.

Myth #1: A glass of red wine a day is good for you.
Wine is sugar. The end. Enjoying the occasional glass of wine or your favorite drink is not the issue when trying to balance hormones—it's more the daily and binge drinking that create hormone chaos. Many women are under the false pretense that a daily glass of wine is "good" for them.

Myth #2: Salads are always nutritious.
Nope. Not if you add a creamy (which usually translates to high-fat) or high-sugar dressing, or you don't vary the ingredients, or if you depend on salads as your only source of fiber. Here's a shocker: the average salad has no more than 5 to 10 grams of fiber. And if you have a weak gut, all that raw food is difficult to digest. Choose steamed veggies or lightly sautéed foods instead.

Myth #3: Green smoothies are always good for you.
I love a good green smoothie, but if you're not careful you can get a sugar boost rather than a fiber or antioxidant burst. The average green

smoothie (store-bought) can have up to 40 grams of sugar and less than 5 grams of fiber. This does not help you reach your hormone goals at all.

If you prep your own green smoothies, use water (not fruit juice) as a base, and make sure your quantity of greens is equal to or greater than your fruit quantity, so you get enough fiber. This will help make your green smoothie work for you, not against you.

Myth #4: Fat makes you fat.
As you have learned, healthy fats don't make you fat; instead, they help build hormones and maintain hormone balance.

Myth #5: Fake sugars help you manage your weight.
False—all those sugar substitutes are really just disrupting your gut bacteria and worsening your inflammation.

Supplement Primer for Hormone Health

"If you're eating well, you don't need to take any supplements." I've lost count of how many patients have told me their doctors have said this to them, downplaying the need for help not just for hormones but also for other issues. This is frustrating, because it's an indisputable fact the nutritional content of our food has declined because our land's soil health is declining. Food no longer contains the nutrient quality it had even twenty-five years ago, and it's only getting worse. Erosion, stripped topsoil, and depleted nutrients are realities of our agricultural times.

Even if you're careful to eat only organic food, it is not necessarily more nutritious—it just is pesticide- and chemical-free. This helps your liver and lowers your toxic load, but it does not guarantee your nutrient tank is filled up.

When your body becomes chronically stressed and nutrient depleted, it goes into triage, figuring out what to keep and what can be sacrificed. High on the sacrifice list are your hormones, particularly estrogen and progesterone. So, this is where supplements can help you feel so much better, assisting your body to build back up what has been depleted and rebuilding the *qi* and prana—your very life force.

This is why one of the cornerstones of Ayurveda and traditional Chinese medicine is the use of herbs, plants, and other substances to treat all kinds of ailments—even those that are hormonal. I use a blended approach, matching nutrient needs with the herbs and supplements that will accomplish the stated goals, relying on the principles of Eastern and Western medicine to bring us back to a natural hormone balance.

Be Supplement Smart: How to Be a Savvy Supplement Consumer

There are countless websites and ads touting the benefits of various supplements, and the claims make it seem as if they will all cure whatever ails you. There's so little regulation of this industry that people are confused what brands are good, what to take, and how much to take. In addition, manufacturers have paid for any testing done, which is often why so few companies do the testing. This is the situation I discovered when I could not find formulas for my patients that blended the best of Eastern and Western medicine. As a result, I launched my own line of supplements, EastWest.

To be supplement smart, you have to know your chemistry. Reading some articles or blogs and grabbing a bottle that's touted as the next big thing, or that your friends use, is not wise. Many of the sales in this enormous industry—the U.S. market was a whopping $35.6 billion in 2022—are for wholly ineffective products. There are many options that are generally considered safe, but too much even of a good thing is not helpful—it can be hard on the liver and harder on the gut. In addition, as you likely know, just because a supplement is available over the counter (OTC) doesn't mean it can't have side effects, especially when combined with other OTC products or prescription medications. It's not necessarily that you're going to hurt yourself, but you're just being inefficient, dancing around an issue instead of targeting it.

Getting supplement smart means learning to read labels. Look at the sourcing of the ingredients. Are they organic, so you know there will be minimal chemical contamination? Where was the product manufactured? Also, are there any certification seals? Bear in mind that certifying organizations like GMP, US Pharmacopeia, NSF International, and ConsumerLab.com test for good manufacturing practices, checking if the products contain what they claim to and aren't contaminated with anything dangerous, like bacteria or lead. Look for these seals on your favorite supplements.

Be sure to check the dosage, too. Some brands are a bit sneaky; you might need to take three or four capsules to get the daily dose, though you bought the product thinking you'd need only one a day.

When you've done your research and found a reputable brand, next thing to do is to prioritize your needs. What is your chief complaint? Is it lack of energy, or interrupted sleep, or moodiness? Focus your supplement choice on one issue at a time, rather than grabbing randomly. That way you'll have a better idea if the supplement will be helpful for you or not. This is the method we use in our clinics, which is a targeted approach, supplementing the key deficiencies after matching those deficiencies to a patient's primary issues and then tracking progress over time and testing regularly. This approach has and continues to work, one patient at a time.

How Long Do Supplements Take to Work?

When my patients tell me about the supplements they're taking, one of the most common complaints is that they haven't seen any results. This may be because the product isn't a good one, or the dosage may not be therapeutic, or it is mismatched to the primary need. There is also an expectation that a supplement will work as quickly as medication, and that simply is not the case.

To judge the supplement's success, at the very least, you should use supplements for at least three weeks, especially if you're dealing with a single issue like energy, sleep, or mood. If you are on the right track, the results are slow but incrementally better, with improvements occurring at three-week, six-week, or three-month intervals.

If you are taking supplements for specific hormone balancing, that will take longer for you to see improvement. Menstruating women need at least ninety days to see any change, because it takes a few monthly cycles for the hormones to adjust and alter what's going on.

The Problem with Supplement Self-Diagnosis

Do you have the BAG?

You know what I'm talking about: the bag that you dump all your supplements into. Picture this: I am getting ready for an appointment, and in walks my patient with the bag. I know what is going to happen next: bottle after bottle is placed on the table, with an anxious patient wanting to know what I think. Was this the right pick? Or this one? Here we go. . . .

I don't recommend self-diagnosis and/or self-treatment for several reasons. First, it's difficult to be objective and it's better to be driven by data. I've made mistakes about my own health because I didn't have the distance and perspective. Second, you want a licensed professional to listen to you, step back, and put the puzzle pieces together, prioritizing your highest needs first.

If you're going to experiment with supplements on your own, without professional support, limit yourself to no more than five different supplements. This might be a vitamin/mineral supplement, magnesium, and a probiotic, for example. Always read the labels to determine the proper dosage, and never exceed the daily dosage. And, as noted earlier, do due diligence when researching brands.

The Most Effective Supplements for Hormone Health

Before you take any supplements, have your vitamin, mineral, and hormone levels checked. You don't want to waste money or risk side effects if you think you're deficient in something when actually you aren't. It's also a good idea to retest if you're on any kind of restrictive diet, have had any recent surgeries, are pregnant, are postpartum, or are dealing with more stress than usual. If any of these are your situation, you'll want to up your supplementation regimen.

Since supplementation is more effective when targeting specific issues, I'm not a huge fan of multivitamin/mineral supplements. They are useful, however, if that's the only supplement you want to take. If so, look for one that contains at least the minimum daily requirement of B vitamins, with antioxidants and iron, because these are the deficiencies most frequently existing in women. If you are sensitive to iron, look for a separate liquid supplement, as it's less likely to cause stomachaches.

Now, let's look at the various forms of supplements.

Vitamin and Mineral Supplements

B vitamins. Look for a methylated B complex supplement containing everything on the following list. If you can't find one, buy them separately.

- B_1: 25 mg (thiamine)
- B_2: 25 mg (riboflavin)
- B_5: 50 mg (pantothenic acid)
- B_6: 50 mg (P5P)
- B_{12}: 1,000 mcg
- Folic acid: 800 mcg
- Biotin: 2,500 mcg

Vitamin D. Take 1,000 IU (international units) of vitamin D_3 daily. (Vitamin D_2 is not well absorbed.) A liposomal formula (encased in a fatlike particle, which makes absorption easier) with at least 100 micrograms of vitamin K will aid effectiveness and absorption.

Calcium. This is needed to maintain strong bones, but several studies have shown that supplements don't decrease the risk of fractures as you get older. Over-supplementation, in fact, leads to a risk for kidney stones and calcification of blood vessels, so it's best to get your daily calcium from foods like fish, greens, dairy, or fortified foods. If you do want to supplement, take no more than 1,000 milligrams per day. Combining calcium with magnesium also enhances absorption. Calcium chelate is the best form to take.

Magnesium. The typical daily dose is 200 to 400 milligrams of chelated magnesium. I've found it helpful to take this before bedtime, as it can ease your getting to sleep. Soaking in a bath with Epsom salts is also a great way to utilize magnesium, as well as to relax your muscles.

Other Supplements and Hormone Boosters

Probiotics. As you learned in Chapter 6, probiotics are an important aid in rebalancing your microbiome. Look for one with at least five different strains of beneficial bacteria and that has at least 50 billion CFU (colony-forming units). Vary the supplement every six weeks or so for an extra boost.

Digestive enzymes. As you also learned in Chapter 6, break your food into smaller pieces so its nutrients are better absorbed. Your supplement should contain amylase (to break down starch), lipase (to break down fat), and protease (to break down protein). It should also have ox bile to better package and metabolize the fats. Since each enzyme is dosed differently, start with one capsule at the heaviest meal of the day. If you have a lot of gas and/or discomfort results, try half a capsule.

Omega-3 fats. These are anti-inflammatories that are also nourishing for your brain and the hormones. They are found in foods like salmon, nut butters, and chia seeds, but getting a high enough supplement dose can be tough. Choose an omega-3 supplement with at least 2 grams of EPA and DHA each.

Adrenal adaptogens. These are herbs that will help balance your adrenal glands and minimize your stress response. Take them before 3 p.m. to help beat the cortisol drops that many women experience in the afternoon. Choose from a daily dose of ashwagandha (1 gram), ginseng (500 milligrams), astragalus (500 milligrams), or licorice root (1 gram).

L-theanine. This is an amino acid that can lower anxiety and improve cognition and focus by increasing the production of the neuro-transmitter GABA. A supplement with 200 milligrams daily is helpful. Anxiety is a primary complaint for women going through hormone swings, so adding this to your list may be helpful.

Choline. This is a phospholipid that helps metabolize fat and regulate insulin, which will improve hormone production in your gut. While it's found in eggs and organ meats like liver, a supplement of 1 gram daily will support your liver, improve insulin resistance, and curb overproduction of androgens as seen in PCOS, perimenopause, and menopause.

Bone broth. This simple liquid has become increasingly popular as a remedy for healing and comfort, although traditional Chinese medicine and Ayurveda have prescribed it for centuries! My mother made it all the time when I was growing up, and I ate it grudgingly, but now I'm grateful that I had such regular goodness, and I do the same thing for my own kids. As the bones simmer, they release nutrients, collagen, and good bacteria, which help you reestablish a healthy gut. Use the best-quality meat or chicken bones you can find. You'll know you've simmered the bones long enough if the water reduces and the broth gels when cooled. Try to drink at least 1 cup (8 ounces) every day.

Supplements to Avoid

I hate to say that a supplement is completely ineffective, because sometimes it might be effective for the right person. Be wary of trends, though, whereby all of a sudden you're seeing umpteen people online touting some product.

I see ads for fat-burning supplements more than just about any other type of supplement. These products often contain caffeine or other ingredients to stimulate the metabolism a little bit, but they're not the answer. Fat burning is about insulin management—so there's no pill to take or tea to drink that will truly burn fat. If there were a fat-burning pill, weight management would be a breeze, wouldn't it?

Here's the bottom line: We all want a quick fix, but no pill is going to change your life. It's the combination of your food and a healthy gut that delivers the nutrient power your body needs for healthy hormones. Know that your chemistry is your own, and you have to do the due diligence to understand it—especially on your Journey UP and as you navigate the hormone shifts.

chapter 8

The Hormonal Laundromat

Our Toxic Environment, Dirty Hormones, and Your Liver

Dirty hormones. Yes, we all have them.

Our environment—food, air, soil, water, homes, skin and body care products—is increasingly toxic. We are facing challenges people did not face a generation ago, and that environment is causing our livers to overwork. The liver is our body's laundromat, taking things in, chopping them up, moving it all to our disposal systems (skin, gut, kidneys, lymphatics, and yes, the liver), so that levels of whatever we've taken in don't build up in the body. This includes hormone metabolites—a.k.a. *dirty hormones*. These dirty hormones actually work against us and can alter our overall hormone balance. High insulin levels, estrogen dominance, high testosterone, high DHT—many of these are caused by dirty hormones, triggering the hormone symptoms and conditions discussed earlier. And the reality is that toxic chemicals are now part of our everyday lives. The toxins you put in or on your body include alcohol, food, drugs, cosmetics, and body care products—and then there are the toxins you inhale from chemicals in your home, cleaners, fragrances, and more. We're finding out that unwanted chemicals are lurking in products we always considered safe. Like baby formula. Water. Indeed, a recent study found that water contaminants once deemed safe are now considered unsafe. Yikes.

Fortunately, you *can* detox your body, and you *can* make your environment and everything in it cleaner. Yes, we do have control—even as our environment changes. And that's the good news. Lowering our toxic load and its burden on our liver is part of the EastWest plan for hormone balancing. And the Thirty-Day Hormone Reset (Chapter 9) tackles this important piece of hormone balancing.

The Spotlight on Your Liver

Finally, this organ of the body is getting the attention it deserves. Think of your liver as the washing machine for your body; it's that important for hormone health.

The liver is the largest internal organ in the body. It needs to be big for a reason—it's responsible for hormonal balance, immune health, and detoxification. In other words, your liver is ground zero for your health. Along with your gut, as I mentioned earlier, it as the laundromat of your body. It takes the toxins, packages them up, and then shoots them out where they can be disposed of.

If the liver and gut can't do their jobs because they are overburdened, you will start to feel it. This distress can be worsened if you have fatty liver syndrome, in which excess body weight leads to insulin resistance and triggers the accumulation of fatty deposits that impede the liver's ability to function properly. If left untreated, inflammation will

The Liver Detoxification Pathways

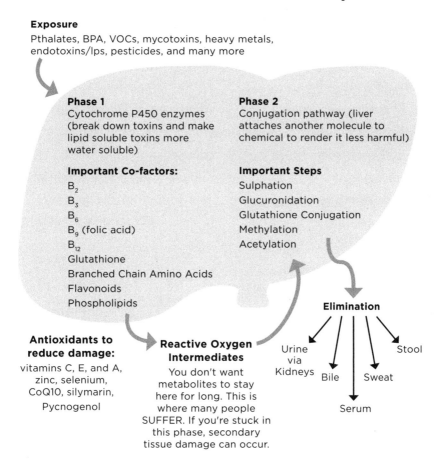

Exposure
Pthalates, BPA, VOCs, mycotoxins, heavy metals, endotoxins/lps, pesticides, and many more

Phase 1
Cytochrome P450 enzymes (break down toxins and make lipid soluble toxins more water soluble)

Important Co-factors:
B_2
B_3
B_6
B_9 (folic acid)
B_{12}
Glutathione
Branched Chain Amino Acids
Flavonoids
Phospholipids

Phase 2
Conjugation pathway (liver attaches another molecule to chemical to render it less harmful)

Important Steps
Sulphation
Glucuronidation
Glutathione Conjugation
Methylation
Acetylation

Elimination
Urine via Kidneys
Bile
Sweat
Serum
Stool

Antioxidants to reduce damage:
vitamins C, E, and A, zinc, selenium, CoQ10, silymarin, Pycnogenol

Reactive Oxygen Intermediates
You don't want metabolites to stay here for long. This is where many people SUFFER. If you're stuck in this phase, secondary tissue damage can occur.

result, along with even more problems such as insulin regulation and hormonal imbalance.

The non-hormonal things that can weigh down your liver go back to the environmental toxins that have been bombarding you through the food you eat, the air you breathe, and the water you drink, as well as aspects of your lifestyle. There can be shocking levels of hidden chemicals in our cleaning products, the products we put on our skin and hair, and the food we eat, as well as the packaging that contains it.

Additionally, hundreds of people die each year, and thousands more go to the emergency room, owing to acetaminophen (Tylenol) toxicity. They didn't realize how dangerous a simple over-the-counter (OTC) painkiller can be for their liver, especially if they drink alcohol at the same time.

If you're super-stressed; if you're taking a lot of conventional Western medications that are metabolized in the liver; if you regularly drink alcohol or eat a lot of sugar—well, the cumulative impact of this environmental load is what traditional Chinese medicine calls *liver blood stasis*, or *liver yang excess*. The liver simply cannot work effectively. It's time to make some changes.

The Phases of Liver Detoxification

For those of you who like to geek out with me, let me explain the two critical pathways for detoxification that take place in the liver.

Phase 1 detoxification. The liver breaks down toxins into particles that can be eliminated from the body. The key nutrients involved in Phase 1 are:

Amino acids

B vitamins

Vitamin A

Vitamin C

Zinc

Phase 2 detoxification. The liver makes the toxins water soluble so they can be sent to the kidneys and the gut, ultimately to be eliminated. The key nutrients involved in phase 2 are:

Amino acids

Glutathione

Molybdenum

Sulfur

Vitamin B$_{12}$

Phase 3 detoxification. This takes place in the cells, where toxins are moved out to—you guessed it—the liver and the kidneys.

More About Dirty Hormones

Dirty hormones, a term I've coined, need to be explained because, if you don't clean them up, it's like you're washing your laundry in dirty water, over and over.

Dirty hormones are the hormone metabolites and hormone by-products that build up in your system as a result of your lifestyle and your genetics, and they cause more harm than good. I discussed them in Chapter 3; they include estrone, 17-hydroxyprogesterone, DHT, derivatives of insulin like fructosamine and high C-peptide, and androstenedione.

If you're feeling off—with symptoms like bloating, breast tenderness, weird rashes, hair loss, and/or acne—chances are high that you have dirty hormones. Often, when these metabolites accumulate, liver toxicity and weight gain are the results. A buildup of dirty hormones activates the genetics for disease. An accumulation of estrogen metabolites, for example, could lead to things like fibroids, breast cancer, endometrial cancer, endometrial hyperplasia, and endometriosis. Further, the metabolites of testosterone or progesterone can act as androgens, making hair loss and acne worse. In fact, I think impaired liver function is partly responsible for increasing cases of precocious puberty, declining fertility, and crossover symptoms such as hair loss, deep voice, and facial hair in women, or gynecomastia and other more estrogen-like traits in men.

The most important thing to understand about dirty hormones is that they're more about hormone *metabolism* than about hormone *levels*. Unfortunately, many doctors get fixated on hormone levels. Let's say you go to your doctor and describe your symptoms, and you're given hormone replacement in the form of estrogen and testosterone. Your hormone levels will correct, and you'll feel like yourself again— but that strategy is treating only the *symptoms*. It's not looking under the hood and saying, "Okay, your estrogen and testosterone levels are much better, but *what is your body doing with them?* Are they getting broken down? If so, are they being eliminated?"

That's why one of the first things I check in all my patients is their hormone metabolites, such as estrone, because most Western doctors don't look for them. This has been an incredibly wonderful and reliable marker for assessments and has helped countless women see where their hormonal imbalances are so they can finally be fixed. Fortunately, once you start addressing your liver's needs and strengthening your gut function (as you'll see in the section on liver detox, pages 258–259), you can clean up your dirty hormones, too.

Quiz: What's Your Toxic Load?

The following quiz will help you understand your own personal toxic load. Take a moment to read these statements, which will help you zoom in on the toxins you are being exposed to. For each item, circle the appropriate response and keep a total of your points.

1. I/We eat out more than two times weekly.

Never (+1)   Sometimes (+3)   Always (+5)

2. I/We buy non-organic produce.

Never (+1)   Sometimes (+3)   Always (+5)

3. I/We buy non-organic meat and/or dairy products.

Never (+1)   Sometimes (+3)   Always (+5)

4. I/We use conventional household cleaners weekly.

Never (+1)   Sometimes (+3)   Always (+5)

5. I/We use standard dry cleaning weekly.

Never (+1)   Sometimes (+3)   Always (+5)

6. I/We use standard insecticides in our home and/or at work.

Never (+1)   Sometimes (+3)   Always (+5)

7. I/We use plastic products to pack lunch or leftovers.

Never (+1)   Sometimes (+3)   Always (+5)

8. I/We grill foods more than once a week.

Never (+1)   Sometimes (+3)   Always (+5)

9. I/We cook with conventional nonstick cookware.

Never (+1)   Sometimes (+3)   Always (+5)

10. I/We use standard bath and/or beauty products.

Never (+1)   Sometimes (+3)   Always (+5)

11. I/We eat cured meats and/or processed cheese.

Never (+1)   Sometimes (+3)   Always (+5)

12. I/We drink alcohol more than three times weekly.

Never (+1)   Sometimes (+3)   Always (+5)

13. I have mercury amalgams (fillings).

Never (+1)   Sometimes (+3)   Always (+5)

14. I watch a plasma TV, or use a cellphone or cordless phone daily.

Never (+1)   Sometimes (+3)   Always (+5)

15. I have more than three to four alcoholic drinks weekly.

Never (+1)   Sometimes (+3)   Always (+5)

Here's an explanation of your results:

0–31

Low toxicity risk. Your toxicity score is low! That's great—keep it up!

32–50

Medium toxicity risk. You have medium risk factors with toxicity. It's time for a tune-up.

51–70

High toxicity score. With a high score, it's time to follow the advice in this chapter as soon as possible.

How Specific Toxins Affect Your Liver

Environmental Toxins

According to the School of Public Health at Tulane University:

Environmental toxins are substances and organisms that negatively affect health. They include poisonous chemicals and chemical compounds, physical materials that disrupt biological processes, and or-

ganisms that cause disease. The effects of exposure to environmental toxins are countless. Major threats include carcinogens, as well as substances affecting cardiovascular, endocrine, and respiratory functions.

The ubiquity of plastics and other synthetic materials, large-scale application of fertilizers and pesticides necessary for industrialized agriculture, the pharmaceutical industry as we know it—all are relatively new. These products have introduced a multitude of chemicals into the environment, and their effects on humans are incredibly complex and largely unknown.

These toxins include pesticides, herbicides, and naturally found substances like blue-green algae, arsenic, mold, and fungi. Pesticides like glyphosate and other organophosphates have been extensively studied and have been shown to impact hormone development, as well as to cause cancers and neurological conditions. Endocrine disrupting chemicals (EDCs) are exogenous chemicals that can contribute to infertility and an increased risk for the development of other hormone-based diseases, including obesity, diabetes, and endocrine cancers.

In addition to outside air pollution, many people have to work in toxic, or sick, buildings. These are buildings with windows that don't open and/or that were built using toxic materials such as asbestos, formaldehyde, and certain plastics. These sealed environments recirculate the same air, day after day. This situation can be exacerbated by exposure to electromagnetic frequencies (EMFs) that impact overall inflammation. This means your computer, your cellphone, and all your other devices may impact toxicity over time.

You also might not know about the environmental toxins in the cleaning products and other household items you have in your home.

Triclosan, for example, is often added to soap and cleansers to make them antibacterial or "odor-fighting," but it's been linked to liver and inhalation toxicity, and even at low levels it can disrupt thyroid function.

And don't get me started about cigarette smoke.

About Xenoestrogens

Xenoestrogens are synthetic estrogens found in the environment (air, water, soil, food) and in products we buy (personal care, cleaning, packaging, birth control pills). Because they are synthetic, they can disrupt normal endocrine functions, leading to dirty hormones.

You wouldn't think that products like fabric softeners and dryer sheets, flea collars, insect repellants, dry cleaning, feminine hygiene products, baby powder, artificial sweeteners, and sunscreen might be harmful. Plastics are one of the worst offenders; you should avoid using plastic containers whenever possible. Never heat up any food in a plastic container, even if it's marked microwave safe.

Skincare and Body Care Products

Who doesn't love the smell, feel, and pleasure that comes from using beauty products? Yet it can be hard to believe that these products used to moisturize your skin and wash your hair can harm your health—but they can. All hair products, makeup, body lotions, and cleansers are absorbed into the skin, which is the largest organ of your body, and your scalp. How do you know what to choose?

I truly do not understand why the U.S. Food and Drug Administration (FDA) is so lax about regulating the toxins in products we put on our bodies every day. In the countries of the European Union, over 1,300 chemicals in cosmetics alone have been banned or restricted. What's the figure for banned chemicals in the United States? *Eleven!*

Cosmetic companies have no legal requirements to test any of their products before they market them. In 2022, for instance, independent testing by the lab Valisure found benzene, a highly carcinogenic chemical, in hundreds of hand sanitizers, sunscreens, deodorants, dry shampoos, hair conditioners, antiperspirants and deodorants, body sprays, and antifungal treatments. The FDA issued a recall for some of the spray products that were so contaminated with benzene that the levels were considered "life-threatening."

Consumers need to do their own due diligence, or risk many of the possible side effects, from minor irritations like rashes to serious health risks like endocrine disruption and cancers. The Environmental Working Group (EWG) can help. They have an excellent, enormous database listing the toxins in everyday products; it can be found at www .ewg.org/skindeep/. In addition, there are helpful apps—such as Think Dirty, GoodGuide, or Apple's Redify—that scan barcodes of your favorite products so you can get their toxicity score.

The Top Ten Toxins Causing Dirty Hormones

How can you gain control and lower your toxic load without going crazy? Here is a list of the top offenders. Read labels, look for these ingredients, and run in the other direction.

Avobenzone. Found in some chemical sunscreens, but while it effectively blocks harmful UV radiation, it paradoxically degrades in the heat of sunlight, releasing harmful free radicals that not only cause aging but increase your risk of cancer. It is also a known endocrine disruptor and is banned for sale in Hawaii (as it also harms coral reefs) and in Europe. Since all sunscreens degrade in the heat, never store them in the bathroom, outside your home, or in your car. A better choice is to use mineral sunscreens only.

BPA, or bisphenol A. A chemical compound found in the lining of aluminum food cans, as well as in plastic bottles, car parts, toys, and even in the paper receipts given to you when you check out in a store. It's a well-known endocrine disruptor, especially as a synthetic estrogen, and has been linked to hormonal irregularities during puberty, heart disease, obesity, diabetes, and cancer.

Formaldehyde or formalin. A key ingredient in most nail polishes and nail products, as well as Brazilian or keratin hair treatments. These chemicals are highly toxic and can cause cancers of the nose, nasal cavity, and throat. They've been linked to cancers, allergies, skin and scalp irritation, hair damage, and hair loss. If you do decide you need a manicure or a hair treatment, make sure the salon is well ventilated. You can buy non-toxic nail polish and bring it to a salon!

Hydroquinone. Used to lighten skin, and because it is cytotoxic, or harmful to cells, it can damage your liver and/or lead to cancer.

Parabens. Chemical preservatives commonly used in many cosmetics and personal care products. Because they mimic estrogen in the body, as such they're a well-known endocrine disruptor that has been linked to breast cancer.

PCBs. Highly toxic chemicals—carcinogenic, endocrine disruptors, and harmful to the immune system—that have been banned in the United States since 1979 but are still found in many areas. They were used in industrial products and in appliances like refrigerators and television sets, and were absorbed into our environment (air, water, and soil) during manufacture and waste disposal, leading to widespread contamination, particularly in landfills, dumps, and the sediment in water sources. It can take many years for PCBs to degrade entirely, and due to this persistence they can be found in fish and seafood, as well as in meat, poultry, eggs, and dairy.

PFAS. Paper take-out containers often contain high levels of fluorine, derived from PFAS, a collection of over 9,000 chemicals used for stain, grease, and water resistance, and in plastic bottles. They're also found in stain- and water-repellents used on carpets, upholstery, and clothing; in cleaning products; in nonstick cookware; and in paints, varnishes, and sealants. PFAS are very dangerous because they don't break down in the environment, and they accumulate in your body. Their presence can affect your reproductive hormones and your thyroid, as well as causing liver, kidney, and developmental problems.

Phthalates. These are industrial chemicals used to make plastics durable or softer. They're found in cosmetics, nail products, shampoos and conditioners, other hair products like hair spray, and soaps, as well as in plastic packaging, garden hoses, vinyl flooring, children's toys, and more. The Centers for Disease Control and Prevention (CDC) has found measurable levels of many phthalate metabolites in the general population, meaning that phthalate exposure is widespread in the U.S. population. This is scary stuff, as phthalates have been linked to allergies, asthma, infertility, endocrine disruption, and insulin resistance.

Phytoestrogens. Naturally occurring bioactive molecules in plants, particularly soy, that mimic estrogen in the body. This makes them a particular risk factor for any woman with an estrogen-receptive cancer.

Triclosan. One of the most commonly added and wholly unnecessary antibacterial agents added to soap and cleansers, triclosan has been linked to liver and inhalation toxicity, and even low levels can disrupt thyroid function.

Alcohol and Toxins

Many people don't realize the intricate relationship between insulin and their liver.

All alcohols are metabolized in the body as sugar, so even one glass of wine will cause an insulin spike and affect your blood sugar level. With a lot of drinking, the liver goes into overdrive to process it all—hence, a hangover. Over time, the more a person drinks, the excess sugar gets converted to fat, which is then stored either in the liver (making it fatty and less productive), in the gut (creating visceral fat, a.k.a. beer belly), or elsewhere in your body. None of this fat is good for you—for your overall health and for your hormones.

Women tend to underestimate how much they can safely drink. The CDC recommends that adults of legal drinking age can choose not to drink or to drink in moderation; that means one drink or less for women in a day or two drinks or less for men. (A drink is 5 fluid ounces [⅔ cup] of wine, 1½ ounces [3 tablespoons] of spirits, or 12 ounces [1½ cups] of beer.) Newer research recommends that both men and women limit their total drinks to under four per week, because the toxic effects of alcohol are becoming more apparent. And I believe that even one drink or less per day for women is still too high when it comes to hormone balance. Factor in the sugar that's found in mixers or juice, and it's no wonder livers are stressed.

For long-term health and prevention, drinking alcohol should be a treat, not a daily habit. Yes, red wine contains the antioxidant resveratrol, and claims have been made that this is good for cardiovascular health. Yet, a study released by the *Journal of the American Medical Association* Network in March 2022 found that there is no level of drinking that does not confer a risk of heart disease. Another study done at the University of Pennsylvania Medical School, included in *Nature Communications* in April 2022, reported that "as drinking increased from one alcohol unit (about half a beer) a day to two units (a pint of beer or a glass of wine) in fifty-year-olds, brain changes were equivalent to the effect of aging two years. An increase from two alcohol units to three showed changes equivalent to aging 3.5 years." This is shocking information; it means that brain volume shrinks, and with it, of course, brain and hormonal function.

In addition, a study by the National Institute on Alcohol Abuse and Alcoholism showed that owing to increased drinking during the isolation of the COVID-19 pandemic, there was a spike of 25.5 percent of alcohol-related deaths in 2020 over the previous year. In 2020, more adults under the age of sixty-five died from alcohol-related factors than from COVID-19.

How to Detox to Help Your Hormones

I hope reading the previous sections of this chapter has made you more determined than ever to reduce your toxic load and give your liver a break. But this can be a overwhelming task, since it feels like something we don't have control over. Fortunately, we do.

Supporting your liver from the inside out will help you achieve the goals of balanced hormones and overall good health. First, you need to fix your internal circuit, then manage your external circuit—your environment, your lifestyle, and your relationships.

Fortunately, your liver, like the rest of your body, *can* regenerate itself to a healthy level. Your body is always striving for balance—a fundamental Eastern concept that also recognizes the body's ability to heal. This is one of the many reasons why you shouldn't give up or tell yourself that you're never going to feel better. Even when damage has been done, you can definitely turn things around and heal over time, even if it's not 100 percent.

How does detoxification work? Your liver, gut, kidneys, lymphatic system, and skin all work together as detoxing agents. Think of it like a five-pointed star. Detoxification is in the middle of that star, with everything else interconnected and acting around it.

The Detoxing Roles of Your Kidneys, Lymphatic System, Gut, and Skin

Your liver isn't the only detoxing organ in your body. Let's consider the other four:

Your kidneys are constantly processing toxins and hormones, but they're doing it through filtration and hydration. Your goal should be to drink 100 ounces (12½ cups) of clean, filtered water daily.

Your lymphatic system is tied to both your immune system and your detoxification pathways, acting as an internal circuit to help move and filter out toxins in the body. A sedentary lifestyle, dehydration, wearing excessively tight-fitting clothing, excessive screen time, and limited sunlight can all slow down lymphatic drainage, further impairing your immune system and increasing the burden on your liver. Exercise, jumping, sweating, massage, and dry brushing are all ways to stimulate your lymphatics.

Your skin is the largest organ of your body and functions as a detoxing organ. Toxins are absorbed into the skin but also excreted through the skin via sweat. Again, exercise, saunas, and whirlpools all help detoxification, partly because of the impact they have on the skin.

Your gut—well, you already know the answer here!

Detox 101

Need a road map for detoxification? Here you go.

Step 1. Your Inner Circuits

Your inner circuitry, a.k.a. your chemistry, is where you begin to think through detoxification. This is the landscape within your control, allowing you to achieve hormone balance and move toxins through your body. Your kidney health, liver, lymphatics, skin, and gut make up this inner circuitry, communicating, weaving together, and doing the work needed to detox.

Step 2. Your External Circuits

Next, you rewire your external circuits, or the influences that operate outside your physical body. Start with your home. What's in your cleaning products? How about the body care products you use every day? Are there long lists of ingredients you don't recognize? Check the EWG to pick brands for cleaning products and body products that minimize the total chemical load and focus on eliminating unnecessary ingredients.

Next, move on to air and water. Ask yourself: What is the quality of the water you drink? Is it from a well or from lead pipes? Do you use a water filter? You can get your water tested or install an infiltration system that filters out many of the chemicals in your drinking water. Indoor air pollution is a rising concern, as well. Opening windows when you're doing any deep cleaning or painting, screening for mold, or off-gassing (chemicals released from paint, cabinets, rugs, some furniture, and wood floors) are initial steps to assess and correct your indoor air quality. There are also devices to measure air quality and many newer, state-of-the-art air filters that help remove these offenders.

Step 3. Food Facts

Eating organic foods is the best way to minimize the toxins found in many food products owing to rampant overuse of pesticides and herbicides, but this can be financially challenging and, if you live in certain small communities, hard to find. Use the EWG's lists (below) of the Dirty Dozen (foods you should try to buy organic) and the Clean Fifteen (foods less likely to be contaminated with pesticides) as a handy guide when shopping. Their lists and much more information are available on their website, ewg.org. If you do buy non-organic items, be sure to wash them thoroughly.

The EWG Dirty Dozen

Strawberries

Spinach

Kale, collards, and mustard
  greens

Nectarines

Apples

Grapes

Bell and hot peppers

Cherries

Peaches

Pears

Celery

Tomatoes

The EWG Clean Fifteen

Avocados

Sweet corn

Pineapples

Onions

Papayas

Sweet peas (frozen)

Asparagus

Honeydew melon

Kiwi

Cabbage

Mushrooms

Cantaloupe

Mangos

Watermelon

Sweet potatoes

While you are becoming familiar with these lists, here are some simple ways to lower your toxic load every day:

- Cut down on alcohol consumption. Goal: under four drinks per week.
- Cut down on sugar. Goal: under 3 teaspoons per day.
- Cut down on foods high in saturated fat, fried foods, and fast food.
- Cut down on items containing food dyes, additives, and preservatives.
- Wash all produce with a food wash (available at grocery stores) to remove pesticides.
- Support farmers by buying fresh organic foods at your local market.
- Grow your own veggies. Even if you live in an apartment in a city, you can grow herbs and items like lettuce in pots on your windowsill.
- If you have vegetable scraps, even onion skins, save them and then throw everything into a large pot to make veggie broth. Strain out the solids and you're good to go. Compost everything else vegetative that might have spoiled.
- Create a food budget and stick to it.

We are living in a culture of overconsumption and waste; we eat too much, buy too much, and then waste too much. We need to flip the mentality of always buying more than we think we need. I learned this during the only trip I've made to India, which was when I was ten years old. My grandmother and aunt and uncle would sit around and chit-chat, and every day it was the same story: *What are we going to cook today?* This became an ordeal for me, because they then had to take me with them to go to all the little shops and fuss over the food. I thought it was the dumbest thing ever. Why couldn't they just buy a few days' worth of food, like my mom did back home?

I used to make so much fun of them, but in hindsight they were right and I was wrong. By buying only what they needed—what was fresh and healthy that day—they weren't over-consuming, overspending, and overeating.

Step 4. House Detoxing

Yes, our world is becoming more toxic, but at the same time there is far more awareness of the toxins found in everyday products. A decade ago, few products claimed to be paraben- or phthalate-free, and now that mention on the label is quite common. It's certainly an important step in the right direction—toward a healthier liver and better hormonal balance.

Refer to the list of the top ten toxins on page 245. Also, with a little bit of scouting, you can find less toxic products that will save you money and avoid liver stress:

- Always use a glass or stainless steel water bottle. Plastic water bottles are a horrible waste of money, as well as terrible for the environment.
- Limit your use of "antibacterial" cleaners with triclosan, fabric softeners and dryer sheets, air fresheners, drain cleaners, oven cleaners, ammonia, bleach, and mothballs.
- Do not use conventional nonstick cookware, as the coatings often contain perfluorooctanoic acid (PFOA), which has been shown to disrupt hormone health. There

are many brands that now manufacture PFOA-free nonstick cookware.

- Use air filters and water filters in your home.
- Biodegradable laundry detergent in sheets can be a better choice than detergents in enormous, nonrecyclable plastic bottles.
- Decorate your house with green plants. They help freshen your indoor air.
- Avoid all use of chemical "air fresheners" with synthetic fragrances, as these increase your exposure to volatile organic compounds, including benzene, toluene, and phthalates.
- If you work in a sick building, one with potential mold, dust, or too much off-gassing (chemicals given off in the environment from paint, floors, fixtures or appliances), take frequent breaks and use a desk-size air filter.
- Use blue screens and blue light blockers on your electronic devices.

How Traditional Chinese Medicine and Ayurveda Tackle Detox

Detoxing Therapies in General

Detoxing is an integral practice in Chinese and Ayurvedic medicine—so much so that they developed a litany of rituals, teas, herbs, and practices to encourage detoxification. These systems also connect emotional health to toxicity. Detoxification is essential to good health in these systems of medicine. This is very different from the eye roll I got from another doctor on a TV appearance, who claimed detoxification is not real.

Traditional Chinese Medicine

The liver meridian in traditional Chinese medicine is a powerful energy channel that dictates everything from detoxification to hormone balance and metabolism. This system also believes that the heat created by stress and anger stays in the liver, so if you are holding a lot of negative feelings, you will wear down the liver energy because the liver meridian is disrupted.

What you should strive to do instead is to calm down and work actively to release those emotions. That's easier said than done, I know, but this book gives you the tools to do exactly this. Your face, tongue, and pulse all tell an emotional story; you will learn more about this in Chapter 9.

I also learned early on in my training in traditional Chinese medicine that deep, uninterrupted sleep is especially crucial for detoxing the liver and lowering the liver "fire," particularly between 1 and 3 a.m. This is the liver meridian's resting time, and if it is interrupted repeatedly, the liver meridian becomes imbalanced. Sleep, therefore, is part of detoxification and is prescriptive for hormone health. This was an Aha moment for me, after years of night shifts and crazy hours—no wonder Hormone Hell was my reality in my twenties!

Ayurveda

Ayurveda is similar to traditional Chinese medicine in the sense that it stresses the importance of gut health and of liver detoxification and support. Herbs and specific diets are often prescribed, and treatments that emphasize body care are essential. Practitioners use mustard oil or sesame oil for vigorous massages. There are seven different types of massage, each having a specific primary function, whether to stimulate lymphatic drainage, move the bowels, or calm the nervous system. The seven types are as follows:

- Abhyangha—stimulation of the internal organs, deep relaxation
- Basti—Joint rejuvenation
- Pizichilli—Elimination of toxins
- Sundarya—Calming facial massage
- Udvartana—Lymphatic drainage, stimulating the metabolism
- Vishesh—Release of deep-seated impurities

And don't forget that yoga is closely tied to Ayurveda, so if you practice yoga even for a short time every day, your liver and your lymphatics (and gut and kidneys) will thank you.

Colonics

When you are constipated and bloated, and you feel like there's toxic sludge sitting in your gut, you might think you need a colonic. This is a treatment whereby a large volume of water is directed into your colon over a period of time, so that what's stuck in there can be removed. Colonics are touted as being a solution to the "toxic waste" in your body, but that is a bit of hyperbole, as they aren't the answer for ridding the body of all its toxins. At best, they are the means for emptying what's been sitting at the end of the colon. If you want to try colonics, limit them to no more than once a month.

My Top Ten Supplements for Detoxing Your Liver

Yes, another Top Ten list! The following product are all helpful in supporting the important work of the liver:

- Calcium D-glucarate—cleanses liver
- Milk thistle—supports liver function
- DIM supplement—breaks down estrogen metabolites
- NAC supplement—glutathione precursor that supports liver health and is a potent antioxidant
- Sesame oil and mustard oil (my mother's favorite)—for softening the skin, easing joint pain, and reducing the toxic load; great to use right out of the shower
- Sulforaphane supplement—made from broccoli sprouts, it improves estrogen detoxification
- Turmeric powder—supports liver health and reduces inflammation
- Jerusalem artichoke—swollen root, used for liver and gallbladder support
- Dandelion root—supplement that serves as a liver cleanser
- Selenium supplement—detoxifies liver

Is It Safe to Do a Liver Cleanse or Detox?

There are countless liver detox programs to choose from, with most giving you a structured plan for three, seven, or ten days, or longer. My first book, *The 21-Day Belly Fix*, features a program to reset your digestive system, and liver detoxification is included, as the liver is considered a digestive organ in Eastern systems of medicine.

A liver detox can be as simple as drinking a plant-based green smoothie for three days in a row, and then adding one or two supplements, like milk thistle or dandelion root, to your daily regimen. Or, it can be as complex as following the advice of a medical specialist to help detox from heavy metals or mold after you've tested positive for exposure.

Please don't start anything more than a simple three-day detox on your own, especially if you have medical issues. Obtain good advice from a credentialed nutritionist or physician. If you're not strong, the detox could cause reactions, such as light sensitivity, rashes, or numbness and tingling in your hands.

Remember, the whole purpose of a detox is to gently rid yourself of toxins and give your liver a break, so if you're having physical reactions, whatever method you are using isn't right for YOU. Find a different plan that won't stress your system.

The Three-Day Detox

If you want a head start on the Thirty-Day Hormone Reset (Chapter 9), this simple three-day detox will be useful for both your body and your mind.

Your Eating Window
1. Create a twelve-hour eating window. For example, eat from 6 a.m. to 6 p.m. or from 8 a.m. to 8 p.m. Keep this up for three days.
2. Wait three to four hours between meals.
3. Stop eating by 9 p.m. every night.

Morning (6–7 a.m.)
1. Drink one apple cider vinegar cocktail upon waking (1 tablespoon vinegar in 3 tablespoons water; never drink vinegar undiluted).

2. Sip 1 cup of warm ginger tea.
3. Eat a brown rice cake with 1 teaspoon coconut oil and
   1 teaspoon olive oil.

Mid-Morning (10 a.m.)

Have a protein shake or smoothie, as snack.

Lunchtime (1 p.m.)

Enjoy a fresh green juice blend.

Mid-Afternoon (3 p.m.)

If you like, have a second green juice blend in mid-afternoon, as a
snack.

Dinner (5–6 p.m.)

Enjoy a dinner of protein and vegetables.

Post-Dinner Snack (7 p.m.)

Have another protein shake or smoothie if you've worked out in
the evening for more than 30 minutes.

Pantry Staples for Your Detox

Have these items on hand before you start the detox:

- Apple cider vinegar (unfiltered organic, such as Bragg
  Organic, Dynamic Health, or Spectrum Naturals)
- Ginger tea (made from 100 percent ginger, such as Alvita
  or Triple Leaf Tea) or homemade from dried or fresh
  ginger

- Brown rice cakes (such as Lundberg Family Farms or Quaker)
- Protein powder (such as Vega One, Metagenics UltraClear Sustain, or Alive Ultra-Shake Pea Protein)
- Coconut oil (virgin or unrefined, such as Spectrum, Dr. Bronner's, or Nutiva)
- Olive oil (extra-virgin, first cold-pressed, such as Olave, Colavita, or Spectrum)
- Frozen unsweetened blueberries
- Frozen mango chunks
- Fresh apples, avocado, bananas, lemons, pears, pineapple; also dried dates
- Fresh vegetables, such as broccoli, carrots, cauliflower, leafy greens, spinach, winter squash, sweet potatoes, zucchini
- Fresh ginger
- Fresh spearmint

As you know by now, the liver plays a major role in hormone balance and hormone health, and it has largely been ignored in conversations about hormones. But when we marry Eastern and Western medicine, managing toxicity prevents dirty hormones, dirty livers, and Hormone Hell, making hormone shifts seamless. It's now time to keep liver health and detoxification at the forefront, as Part III begins and we learn about the Thirty-Day Hormone Reset. Let's begin your Journey UP!

The Journey UP: Resetting Your Hormones

chapter 9

The Thirty-Day Hormone Reset

Are you ready? Ready to find hormone balance, energy, and, most important, your oomph? You have come to understand the many nuances of Hormone Hell and the hormone shifting that is natural for all women—and you are ready to take ownership of that journey. It's your Journey UP.

I am thrilled to boost you on your way to success. Sure, it's about getting your chemistry right, but it's also about your realizing the fullest expression of yourself: your gifts, talents, and purpose, finally revealed and working in synergy with the rest of you. We address all of this in this chapter.

Prep Work

Where to start? The Thirty-Day Hormone Reset begins with a bit of prep work to establish a solid foundation for hormone-healthy habits. As a busy woman, you know that staying organized, with everything easily accessible, makes your goals more attainable. So, let's begin with some simple tasks.

Kitchen Cleanup

We often spend the most time in our day in the kitchen. Food is our first medicine, but to make it work for you in your busy life, you have to be organized. The Thirty-Day Hormone Reset calls for a change in your eating patterns, and to make this change successful, it has to be easy. In the spirit of simplification, take a day to "trash and stash" your kitchen items, as follows:

TRASH	
Bacon	Bleached white flour
Canned fruits	Canned soups, full-sodium broths
Canned vegetables	Condensed milk
Desserts	Fat-free dairy products
Fat-free dressings	Flavored yogurts
Food dyes (all colors)	High-fructose corn syrup (or products with it, including ketchup, pancake syrup)
Margarine	Packaged or convenience foods (chips, crackers)
Powdered dip mixes	Pre-made gravy
Processed peanut butter	Seasoned coatings and breadcrumbs
Splenda sugar substitute	Sausages
Vegetable oils (soybean, corn)	White (granulated) sugar

Whole Grains	Amaranth, quinoa Barley Brown rice, wild rice Couscous Kamut Millet Steel-cut oats Rye Spelt
Fresh and Frozen Fruit and Vegetables	
Healthy Oils and Fats	Avocado oil Coconut oil Ghee (clarified butter) Grapeseed oil Olive oil Safflower oil Sunflower oil
Sauces and Condiments	Avocado sauce, guacamole Barbecue sauce, free of high-fructose corn syrup Hot sauce Hummus Ketchup, unsweetened Lemon juice Liquid aminos Mustard Pasta sauce, unsweetened, low sodium Pesto Red pepper sauce Salsa Tamari Tomatillo sauce Tomato paste, tomato sauce Vinegar
Dairy and Non-dairy	Cottage cheese Farmer cheese Kefir Milk, full-fat, or coconut, almond, oat Paneer Ricotta cheese Yogurt, Greek

Spices and Fresh Herbs	Basil Black pepper Cayenne Cilantro Cumin Garlic, garlic powder, garlic salt Ginger (ground and fresh) Lemon pepper Oregano Parsley Paprika Salt Turmeric (powder and root)
Drinks	Fruit water Herbal teas Vegetable juices Water, still or sparkling
Protein	Beans (navy, pinto, black, garbanzo, kidney) Beef/pork, lean Chicken Eggs Fish Goat Lentils Nut butters
Breads and Pasta	Brown rice pasta Buckwheat pasta Chickpea pasta Lentil pasta Sprouted grain bread (such as Ezekiel) Sourdough, whole-grain, or gluten-free bread

Bedroom Basics

A cluttered bedroom, a TV constantly on, computers running, and cellphones in use—none of these promotes a healthy night's sleep or provides a sanctuary where the mind can rest. Remove unnecessary clutter from your bedroom, move out the computers, place the cellphone at least six feet away from where you sleep, and create a small space for you to meditate, write, pray, or just get inspired. Your space should reflect who you are, with the colors, textures, and tones that make you happy. Add your favorite essential oils, perhaps speakers for relaxing music, or even a sound bath, and pick out your favorite sheets, blankets, and pillows. This is your sanctuary—make it look like one.

Cellphone/WiFi Rules

It's time to get disciplined about the devices. And yes, I sound like your mom, but these are your doctor's orders; it's one, to be completely honest, that I struggle with myself. Here are the rules:

1. No checking email or social media just before you go to bed. Instead, head to your sanctuary.
2. At night, put your phone on dark or grayscale mode. This lowers the dopamine response you get when constantly going to your phone.
3. Place blue light blockers on your devices to lower the amount of electromagnetic frequency you are exposed to.
4. Put the phone away thirty minutes prior to bedtime.

What in the world do these rules have to do with your hormones? *Everything.* The quality of your sleep, your food, and amount of stress you feel all control your hormones, perhaps keeping you in a toxic-hormone state; it's that toxic state that makes you feel and look like that stranger in the mirror.

There's a large chunk of time when your body is talking to you but you are just not listening—until the crash. Why do we all wait that long? I wish we could wear a sensor that would alert us when our systems are starting to fail, like the gas gauge in a car or the smoke alarm in your home. That might get us to be more self-aware, right? But until that invention hits the market, there are vital signs you can track as you move through the Thirty-Day Hormone Reset, helping you understand and decode your body's language.

The Vital Signs

Most people hear the words *vital signs* and assume those that are taken in the doctor's exam room or in a hospital—assessing our temperature, pulse, heart rate, oxygen level, and blood pressure. But our vital signs are evident everyday—every moment, in fact—and they can educate us on our mental, physical, and emotional states.

As you move through the Thirty-Day Hormone Reset, you will track the following vital signs. By doing so, you will start to understand what your body is saying to you, and you will have data points to guide you as to what's working and what may need to be tweaked.

Vital Sign	Goals	Increased	Decreased
Resting heart rate (RHR)	60–75 bpm	High cortisol, high insulin	Hypothyroid, malnutrition
Heart rate variability	40–60 ms	Better cortisol balance, better overall stress response	High cortisol, high stress, high insulin, cardiovascular disease
Blood pressure (BP)	100/60–120/80	High cortisol, estrogen dominance, hyperthyroid	Malnutrition, depletion
Basal body temperature (BBT)	97–97.5°F	Higher progesterone, low estrogen ovulation, pregnancy, hyperthyroidism, infection	Hypothyroidism, fatigue, weight gain, estrogen excess

Tracking these numbers can help you understand how you are responding to the plan or where you might be at this moment, the very beginning. If, for example, your resting heart rate is high and your heart rate variability is low, you may be in a more stressed state. Significantly low blood pressure and low basal body temperature are associated with a more sluggish thyroid or being low in protein and key nutrients.

Many of my patients also use glucometers to measure blood sugar, as well as Oura rings or WHOOP bands to track the quality of their sleep. Many Apple watches and Fitbit trackers are also tracking sleep patterns, but even just charting how often you wake up at night and if you feel refreshed in the morning is easy. These are also helpful data points, forcing us all to reckon with the days we are super-stressed, depleted, or have shifting hormone levels.

Lastly, don't forget that checking your tongue, reading your face, and assessing where you are on the emotional spectrum (as described in Chapter 4) provide additional tools to assess your overall state of being. I recommend tracking all these data points at least weekly and then reflecting on what could have influenced the numbers or your answers. The chart on page 272 will help you track the data.

Navigating Your Hungers—Wants vs. Needs

Last but not least, how do you recognize the signs of true hunger versus stress eating? Most people aren't really hungry anymore, and we wouldn't even recognize true hunger, because we have so many stores of fat we can use if needed, especially as people have gotten used to enormous portion sizes. When I was growing up, a cup of coffee was no more than 6 or 8 ounces (³⁄₄ to 1 cup), a glass bottle of Coke was a mere 6½ ounces (³⁄₄ cup), and a serving of pasta was not even 2 ounces.

Stress eating is different; we've replaced what we're feeling with the sensation of hunger. I agree with experts who say that much of what we think of as hunger is not a physical state, it's an *emotional* one. It's a feeling of deprivation, a feeling of lack, a feeling of want—but it's not necessarily a clue that we need to eat. So, it's up to you to identify your feelings when you think hunger pangs are pinging and decide whether to pay attention to that signal or not. This is why some people, when they are stress eating, tend to want comfort foods. For some people, the comfort food is crunchy; for others, it's sweet or chewy. And some of those cravings are related to hormone imbalances, too.

To make it easier for you to know when to eat, I devised a system that I call *biorhythmic eating*. It sounds a bit like a dance, doesn't it? It actually is a bit of a dance as we're moving right along with our hormones. Their release doesn't follow a straight line; we're on a curvy line constantly.

What you're looking for with biorhythmic eating is awareness. *Mindfulness* is awareness. Many nutritionists suggest that women wanting to lose weight or be more mindful of their eating habits keep a food diary. I don't think that's the best suggestion for two reasons. One is that it's easy to forget to do this if you have a busy day. The other is that if you're eating foods that aren't healthy for you, there can be a lot of shame involved, so you don't include them on your list, and that is never helpful.

Instead, you follow your own rhythm. Just as we have circadian rhythms that regulate our sleep/wake cycle, we each have a unique hormonal biorhythm.

One way to look at this is that our bodies are basically running on a comprehensive, interconnected chemical circuit, which is our biorhythm. It's hard to say where the actual starting point of this circuit is because the hypothalamus and the pituitary gland are located in your brain, signaling to different organs when to release their hormones. At the same time you've got all the different organs secreting some kind of hormone as we saw in in Chapter 3. Everything from your ovaries, your liver, your kidneys, your pancreas, your bones, your tissues, your skin, your muscles— all of them are endocrine organs that should be functioning and working together in an endless loop of hormone release and hormone synthesis.

There's also another circuit, which is our lifestyle—whether it's diet, stress, sleep, toxins, relationships, trauma—all the aspects of daily life.

Your lifestyle biorhythm influences the chemistry component of your hormonal biorhythm. Any of your lifestyle factors can block the circuit. This is akin in a way to traditional Chinese medicine, where your *qi* flows along an invisible circuit inside your body, and when it gets stuck in certain meridians, the use of acupuncture needles can unblock the *qi*.

When your hormones are imbalanced, it's almost like you're tripping your own circuits in your body, and that impacts your body map, or the place where the five bodies (mental, physical, emotional, energetic, and social) intersect. These symptoms of imbalance have been discussed in earlier chapters, so you know how they impact your mental health, sleep, social life, and overall energy. The circuits get restarted when the hormonal balance is restored, returning health and wellness to all five bodies. This central concept of biorhythms and interconnectedness is why you can't just use weight training without also improving your nutrition, and you can't scarf down supplements but skimp on sleep. You can't improve your overall health without going to the root causes of your issues and treating your body as a whole.

This is why the eating component of hormonal balance is so important. Your hormonal biorhythm is a new way to think about why and when you're eating. It will help you eat only when you're hungry, put nutrient-rich food into your body, and minimize your hormone conditions at the same time.

Okay, the prep work is over. It's time to get down to the business of hormone balancing. It may help to read through the entire plan first to get the lay of the land. At the end, there's a quick-reference outline you can use as a road map. Here we go: for the next thirty days, you'll be resetting your hormones and yourself.

PHASE 1

Days 1–7

Minding Your Mitochondria and Reversing Oxidative Stress

Do you know what so many women tell me every day in practice? That they are tired—utterly exhausted, and they simply cannot get through their day. That fatigue may be emotional, cognitive, or physical, but at some point it becomes debilitating.

There are so many places to potentially initiate a hormone reset, but we start with the Eastern concept of building *qi*, or energy. In integrative and functional medicine, this translates to minding the mitochondria, which is the powerhouse of the cell, and in replenishing nutrients. As cells become nutrient depleted, oxidative stress sets in, meaning the cells are deprived of oxygen and slowly die, leaving the body depleted and tired.

Yep, we have to refill the tank, so to speak, to have the energy even to carry out any plan of any kind. If you got tired doing the prep work, then this first phase of the reset may be the most important one of all. You simply must rebuild your *qi*.

Tactically, this means you need nutrients, water, protein, and sleep. In traditional Chinese medicine, these all provide energy: broths to heal the gut and increase iron and protein, herbs to lower cortisol, and lots of rest. In fact, the ancient Greek physician Hippocrates would put patients in an underground sleep chamber to force them into a healing state. But we are living in the second millennium, so sleep chambers and lots of broth may be out of the question. Instead, let's find a more realistic way to build energy.

Step 1. Add One 6-Ounce Green Smoothie Daily

Green smoothies are an easy way to increase your stores of glutathione, a potent antioxidant that powers the mitochondria, rejuvenating the liver, brain, and heart, and reducing inflammation. Note that green smoothies are different from green juices; you want to keep the fiber so that there is not a massive spike in blood sugar levels. And fresh green smoothies have been found to have a lot of glutathione and additional antioxidants (vitamins A, C, and E, and CoQ10), all needed for healthy hormone balance.

Choose from one of the recipes below or have fun on your own.

Basic Green Smoothie
MAKES 1 SERVING

1 cup chopped seasonal greens
$^1/_4$ cup chopped frozen fruit
$^2/_3$ to $^3/_4$ cup water, fresh juice, or non-dairy milk
1 banana or avocado

Place the ingredients in a blender and process until smooth.

Liver Lover's Smoothie
MAKES 1 SERVING

1 cup chopped raw or steamed beets
1 medium carrot, coarsely chopped
1 celery stalk, coarsely chopped
$^1/_2$ cup dandelion greens
$^1/_4$ cup fresh parsley
$^1/_4$ cup fresh cilantro
$^3/_4$ to 1 cup water (or ice)

Place all the ingredients in a blender and process until smooth.

Green Green Smoothie

MAKES 1 SERVING

2 cups fresh spinach

1 ripe pear, cored and chopped

15 seedless grapes

1 (6-ounce) container coconut yogurt

2 tablespoons chopped ripe avocado

Squeeze of lime juice

Place the ingredients in a blender and process until smooth.

Fruity Delight Smoothie

MAKES 1 SERVING

1 cup stemmed and chopped fresh kale

$\frac{1}{2}$ cup frozen cherries

$\frac{1}{4}$ cup frozen blueberries

1 cup water

Place the ingredients in a blender and process until smooth.

Step 2. Add High-Glutathione Foods

This step is about learning more hormone-powering food substitutions. Switching out some of the ingredients in your favorite recipes to the ingredients below is another way of boosting your internal stores of glutathione. Adding more high-glutathione foods to your diet helps to support mitochondrial health and improve overall energy. Try to have two servings daily—a serving is about $\frac{1}{2}$ cup or 3 ounces for meats. A few examples include:

Asparagus	Beets	Brown rice	Chicken
Beef	Broccoli	Cauliflower	Eggs

| Fish | Kale | Spinach |
| Garlic | Lentils | |

If you love iceberg lettuce in your salads, for example, switch to kale or spinach. Add garlic where you can to dressings and marinades. Or swap out white rice for brown rice. However you do it, adding two servings daily of any of the items above to your breakfast, lunch, or dinners helps build your *qi*.

Step 3. Up the Protein

I find that many women are tired simply because they are not getting enough protein—protein powers the mitochondria, preserves muscle mass, and keeps blood sugar stable. Protein provides the amino acids to power up our cells, building energy. Additionally, hormone balancing is connected to blood sugar balance (remember insulin), and when we look at the science, 20 to 30 grams of protein in any form, every three to four hours, achieves blood sugar stability. This translates to one to two scoops of a protein powder (depending on the brand), 3 to 4 ounces of lean meats or fish, and approximately 1⅓ cups of most cooked beans. (See protein sources table on page 219.) You can add a few scoops of protein powder to oatmeal or baked goods as well, or just whip up your favorite smoothie. During your hormone reset, you can add the protein into your green smoothie, or you can start your day with a protein smoothie, then follow up with the green smoothie for a boost of energy about two hours later. Protein powders or supplements include those from brown rice, eggs, hemp, mixed plants, and peas.

Here are a few of my favorite protein-powered morning breakfasts:

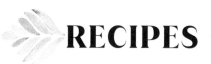

RECIPES

Four Protein Smoothies

Chocolate Protein Smoothie
MAKES 1 SERVING

    1 ripe banana (or frozen, for thicker texture)
    2 scoops (about 20 grams) protein powder
    1 tablespoon nut butter of choice
    1 heaping tablespoon semisweet mini chocolate chips (stevia sweetened,
        if available)
    1 cup unsweetened almond or coconut milk

Place all the ingredients in a blender and process until smooth.

Skinny Mocha-Banana Jump-Start
MAKES 1 SERVING

    1 frozen banana
    $\frac{1}{2}$ cup cold coffee (or 1 teaspoon instant coffee)
    1 to 2 scoops (20 grams) chocolate protein powder (see Note)
    1 cup rice, cashew, or unsweetened coconut milk

Place all the ingredients in a blender and process until smooth.

Note: For additional protein, add nut butters, ground flax seed, or collagen powder.

Pumpkin Power Smoothie

MAKES 1 SERVING

 $1/2$ cup canned pumpkin puree

 1 medium apple, cored and sliced

 1 cup milk of choice

 $1/2$ cup ice cubes, plus more if desired

 $1/4$ cup plain yogurt (plant-based, if desired)

 1 to 2 scoops (20 grams) vanilla protein powder

 1 teaspoon vanilla extract

 1 teaspoon pumpkin pie spice (mix of cinnamon, nutmeg, ginger, cloves, and allspice)

Place all the ingredients in a blender and process until smooth.

Mint Chip Smoothie

MAKES 1 SERVING

 $1/4$ cup unsweetened coconut milk

 $1/4$ cup Greek yogurt (or coconut yogurt, for dairy-free)

 1 frozen banana, chopped

 2 cups fresh spinach

 1 to 2 scoops (20 grams) vanilla protein powder

 $1/2$ teaspoon vanilla extract

 $1/2$ teaspoon peppermint extract, or as desired

 1 tablespoon chopped 85% dark chocolate (or stevia-sweetened mini chocolate chips)

 Water, as needed

Place all the ingredients in a blender and process until smooth.

Protein Overnight Oats

MAKES 1 SERVING

$\frac{1}{2}$ cup gluten-free old-fashioned rolled oats

$\frac{3}{4}$ cup unsweetened vanilla almond milk

1 to 2 scoops (20 grams) vanilla protein powder

$\frac{1}{2}$ tablespoon chia seeds

$\frac{1}{2}$ teaspoon vanilla extract

$\frac{1}{4}$ teaspoon ground cinnamon

1 tablespoon nut butter

$\frac{1}{3}$ cup chopped fresh fruit, such as peach, pear, blueberries, raspberries, strawberries

Place the oats, almond milk, protein powder, chia seeds, vanilla, and cinnamon in a pint container or glass jar, shake, cover with a lid, and place in fridge overnight.

Remove the jar from the fridge in the morning and stir. Scoop into a bowl. (Note: The oatmeal and chia seeds will be thick, having soaked up most of the liquid. If you prefer a thinner consistency, add some water or almond milk to reach your desired consistency.)

Stir in the nut butter and sprinkle the fruit on top.

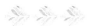

Step 4. Add Energy-Boosting Supplements

You are still building energy this week, so adding in a few supplements to help boost mitochondrial function can provide energy to depleted cells and prep you for the next few weeks of the plan. Consider taking the following supplements.

Methylated B vitamins

A B-complex vitamin containing methyl B_{12}, methyl folate, and P5P (pyridoxal-5-phosphate) is important for the metabolism and detoxification of hormones, as well as for overall energy. This is one of the most common deficiencies I find in women. Look for a supplement with at least 1,000 micrograms (μg) of methyl B_{12}, 800 micrograms (μg) of methyl folate, and 25 milligrams of P5P.

NAC

N-acetyl cysteine is an intermediate of glutathione and is absorbed orally. Consider taking 500 milligrams per day to start. If you have sulfur allergies, try the Ayurvedic herb powders shatavari and amla instead (1 gram of each).

Step 5. Maintain a Consistent Sleep Cycle and Keep a Twelve-Hour Overnight Fast

Sleep is the foundation of energy, and we can't get too much further in the plan without evaluating your sleep quality. It's important to maintain a consistent sleep pattern. In Chinese medicine, women ideally sleep between 11 p.m. and 5 a.m., as this part of the circadian rhythm determines hormone balance. I want you to aim for at least eight hours. You can set your own schedule—for example, 11 p.m. to 7 a.m. or 10 p.m. to 6 a.m. Try your utmost to follow this pattern at least four nights per week. If you are a shift worker, perhaps try to batch your shifts in three-day stints, with four days each week for recovery.

At the same time, we are going to prep to start following a more anti-inflammatory, insulin-balancing eating plan that benefits everyone. The first step is to keep a twelve-hour overnight fast; meaning, for example, if you stop eating at 8 p.m., don't eat again until 8 a.m. This period of fasting allows for overnight gut rest and improves digestion.

If you are having trouble sleeping, I recommend adding in magnesium 200 milligrams nightly or herbs to help with staying asleep, including any one of the following:

Holy basil: 500 milligrams
Ashwaghandha: 500 milligrams
Magnolia bark: 500 milligrams

HORMONE RESET

Days 8-15

Gentle Detox and Inflammation Reduction

By this point, you are likely feeling better. You have more bandwidth and more energy. This is a good time to check your vital signs, take a look at your tongue, and consider where you are along the emotional spectrum. You should have taken a step up and are now ready for some serious cleanup.

The next seven days of the Thirty-Day Hormone Reset address the powerhouses and home of hormone balance: the gut and the liver. In Eastern systems of medicine, these are both part of the digestive system, and they need to be balanced and cleaned before moving on to the hormone nitty-gritty. A healthy gut and liver reduce inflammation and improve your body's detoxification capacity, allowing hormones to be used the right way. And as we have discussed, we cannot do any form of hormone replacement until these two organs are working well.

The gut and liver rehab program does not have to be painful or high maintenance, but it does need to happen. Here is what you do next: continue steps 1 through 5 of Phase 1 (pages 276–282).

Step 6. Remove All Inflammatory Foods

Yes, we are getting serious. Now that you've built up your energy level, you can get pickier about the foods you eat and make sure that your diet is serving you. You may already know that particular foods trigger an inflammatory response, so keep them out of your kitchen or track your vital signs after trying them. For the next three weeks, you will be taking out the inflammatory foods appearing in the following list. These are the heavy hitters:

Alcohol

Dairy

Gluten

Processed meats

Processed soy products

Sodas

Sugar

Trans fats (found in packaged goods)

White bread

White-flour pasta

Instead, add these hormone-healthy foods—you may recognize some of these on our glutathione foods list.

Chicken or turkey

Fish and other seafood

Fresh vegetables

Fruits

Lean beef

Legumes

Nuts

Seeds

Sparkling water

Whole grain, seeded, or sprouted breads

This is your week to continue to look at your food choices and swap out for hormone-healthier options. Maybe trade the nightly alcohol for sparkling water, dairy for nut butters, and processed meats for grilled chicken, cauliflower, or grass-fed beef. The recipes below remove inflammatory foods while still providing the protein and mito foods we need for healthy hormones. You can use these recipes as laid out or mix and match for breakfast, lunch, or dinner.

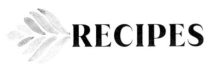

RECIPES

Two Anti-inflammatory Breakfast Choices

Tofu Scramble

MAKES 2 SERVINGS

1 tablespoon coconut oil or ghee (clarified butter)

1 tablespoon chopped red onion

1 (14-ounce) package extra-firm tofu, cut into small squares

1 cup chopped fresh kale, spinach, or Swiss chard

1 ripe tomato, chopped

$^1/_2$ teaspoon Himalayan or table salt

$^1/_2$ teaspoon paprika

Pinch of ground black pepper

2 tablespoons crumbled feta or chèvre

In a skillet, melt the oil over medium-high heat. Cook the onion, stirring frequently, for 2 minutes, until tender. Add the tofu and cook, stirring frequently, until lightly browned, about 3 minutes. Add the greens and tomato and cook, stirring, for 1 to 2 minutes, until the greens are wilted and the tomato has softened. Stir in the salt, paprika, and pepper.

Divide the mixture between two plates. Sprinkle each with the cheese and serve.

Egg and Veggie Wrap

MAKES 1 SERVING

1 teaspoon coconut oil, ghee (clarified butter), or olive oil

1 tablespoon diced yellow onion

$^1/_2$ cup chopped fresh spinach or kale leaves

2 large eggs

$^1/_2$ teaspoon paprika

Salt and black pepper

1 gluten-free wrap or corn (or gluten-free) tortilla

Heat a medium skillet over medium heat. Add the oil and heat until it shimmers. Add the onion and cook until translucent, about 3 minutes, then add the greens and cook until wilted, 2 to 3 minutes.

In small bowl, whisk the eggs, then add to the skillet, scrambling them as they cook in the spinach. Add the paprika and salt and pepper to taste.

Place the wrap on a serving plate. Spoon the egg-spinach mixture on it and close the wrap.

Three Anti-inflammatory Lunch Ideas

Broccoli Salad with Tahini Sauce

MAKES 2 SERVINGS

6 cups finely chopped broccoli (from 3 to 4 large crowns)

$\frac{1}{2}$ cup minced red onion

1 medium cucumber, chopped

$\frac{1}{2}$ cup fresh parsley, chopped

2 tablespoons hemp seeds

Juice of 1 large lemon

5 tablespoons tahini paste

3 tablespoons water

3 tablespoons olive oil

1 garlic clove, minced

Salt and black pepper

Quickly blanch and drain the broccoli. Place in a large bowl and add the onion, cucumber, parsley, and hemp seeds.

In a small bowl, combine the lemon juice and tahini paste and whisk with a fork, adding the water slowly as you mix. When the sesame paste is dissolved, it should coat the back of a spoon. Pour in the olive oil and garlic, then season to taste with salt and pepper.

Pour the dressing over the broccoli mixture and toss well. Let rest in the fridge for 30 minutes to 1 hour before serving to let the flavors develop.

For additional protein, add in 1 egg, 1 tablespoon nut butter, or 7 ounces tofu.

Stir-Fried Zoodles with Creamy Satay Sauce

MAKES 2 SERVINGS

- 3 medium zucchini or summer squash
- 6 to 8 ounces diced raw chicken, beef, or shrimp (optional)
- 1 tablespoon oil (optional; can be olive, avocado, or grapeseed)
- 1 garlic clove, minced
- 3 to 4 tablespoons nut butter (cashew or almond work best)
- 2 tablespoons tamari or gluten-free soy sauce
- 1 tablespoon toasted sesame oil
- 1 teaspoon honey
- $\frac{1}{2}$ teaspoon red pepper flakes, or more if desired
- $\frac{1}{4}$ teaspoon Chinese five-spice powder (fennel seeds, ground peppercorns, anise, cloves, cinnamon; optional)
- 1 cup chopped napa cabbage or red cabbage
- $\frac{1}{4}$ cup chopped red onion or scallion whites
- Lime slices or minced cilantro, for serving

If possible, spiralize the zucchini (or slice it with a mandoline) and press out excess water with a paper towel. Set aside.

Heat a large skillet to medium heat. If using the chicken, beef, or shrimp, add the oil to the pan, and then add the protein, stirring and turning until cooked through, about 8 minutes; the shrimp will take slightly less time. Remove from the pan and set aside.

In the same skillet, add the garlic, nut butter, tamari, sesame oil, honey, red pepper flakes, and five-spice powder. Heat, stirring, until combined and creamy, about 3 minutes.

Toss in the cabbage and onion and stir-fry for 2 minutes, until both are softened. Add the zucchini and protein, if using. Stir-fry 1 more minute, until the zucchini noodles are coated with sauce but still firm.

Transfer to plates and garnish with lime or cilantro.

Build-Your-Own Buddha Bowl

VARIABLE SERVINGS

Here's a four-step construction of a healthy bowl you can prepare and serve any number of people. In a large bowl, layer in *healthy carbohydrates*: chopped sweet potato, cooked quinoa, brown rice, barley, rice noodles. Add the *veggies*: sliced or spiralized zucchini or summer squash, fresh spinach, grated carrots, sliced red or green cabbage, bell peppers, cucumber, avocado, steamed peas, chopped kale, some leaves of romaine lettuce, radish slices. Stir in the *protein*: nuts, seeds, cooked lentils or beans, organic tofu, shrimp, chicken, grass-fed beef.

Prepare your *sauce*: use your favorite dressing, or try something new, like an avocado aioli or a cilantro-lime sauce. Pour the sauce over the ingredients in the bowl.

If desired, add *garnishes*: chopped fresh cilantro, grated onion, sesame seeds, crushed nuts, hemp seeds, sunflower seeds.

If you are unsure about amounts, see my Protein Guide on page 219.

Four Anti-inflammatory Dinner Choices

Sautéed Fresh Greens with Sweet Potato and Turkey

MAKES 3 OR 4 SERVINGS

Olive oil, for cooking
1 pound ground turkey, crumbled
1 medium sweet potato, cut into 1-inch cubes
2 cups mixed fresh kale, chard, spinach, and/or dandelion greens
1 tablespoon minced onion
1 garlic clove, minced
Salt and black pepper

Heat a large skillet over medium-high heat, then add a drizzle of olive oil to coat the pan. When the oil is simmering, add the ground turkey and cook until lightly browned and cooked through, stirring to break up any clumps, about 10 minutes. Transfer the turkey to a bowl and set aside.

Turn down the heat to medium-low and add another drizzle of oil. Add the sweet potato, greens, onion, and garlic. Cover the skillet with a lid and let the greens and potatoes steam for 7 to 10 minutes, until the potatoes are soft and the greens are wilted.

Add the turkey to the skillet again and stir to combine. Season to taste with salt and pepper, then serve immediately.

Secret Kale Salad

MAKES 2 SERVINGS

1 bunch fresh kale, stemmed and leaves sliced into small strips

Zest and juice of 1 lemon

$\frac{1}{4}$ cup olive oil or avocado oil

1 garlic clove, minced

Pinch of Celtic, Himalayan, or sea salt

2 teaspoons honey

$\frac{1}{4}$ cup unsweetened dried cranberries

$\frac{1}{4}$ cup pine nuts or sunflower seeds (or a combination)

Place the kale strips, lemon zest and juice, oil, garlic, and salt in a large bowl. With your hands, massage the kale strips with the other ingredients for about 2 minutes to soften (this is the secret behind delicious kale salads).

Add the honey, cranberries, and nuts. Toss to combine well. Let the salad rest for 15 to 20 minutes to meld the flavors before serving.

For protein additions, see the Protein Guide on page 219 for ideas.

Tandoori-Spiced Salmon with Yogurt-Cucumber Sauce

MAKES 2 SERVINGS

SALMON

1 (4- to 6-ounce) salmon fillet

Cooking spray

$\frac{1}{2}$ lemon

$\frac{1}{2}$ cup plain Greek yogurt

2 teaspoons tandoori spice mix or ground red pepper

1 teaspoon ground turmeric

1 teaspoon curry powder

$\frac{1}{4}$ teaspoon salt

4 garlic cloves, mashed with a little water to make a paste

1 teaspoon ginger paste (or puree 1 teaspoon minced fresh ginger with water to create a paste)

1 tablespoon olive oil

YOGURT-CUCUMBER SAUCE

1 cup plain Greek yogurt

1 small cucumber, finely chopped

$\frac{1}{2}$ teaspoon chopped fresh parsley

$\frac{1}{2}$ teaspoon chopped fresh cilantro

Preheat the oven to 350°F.

Prepare the salmon: Rinse the fish and pat it dry with paper towels. Coat a small baking pan with cooking spray, then arrange the fish in the pan. Squeeze the lemon half over the fish.

In a small bowl, combine the yogurt, tandoori spice, turmeric, curry powder, salt, garlic paste, and ginger paste. Mix well to make a smooth paste.

Brush the salmon with the olive oil. Spread the paste liberally on both sides of the fillet. Return the to the pan and cover with foil. Bake for 15 minutes.

Meanwhile, make the yogurt sauce: In a small bowl, combine the yogurt, cucumber, parsley, and cilantro. Mix well until smooth.

Finish the salmon: Remove the foil and turn the oven to broil. Broil the fish for 2 to 3 minutes, until lightly browned on top. Serve with the yogurt-cucumber sauce.

Faux Fried Coconut Chicken with Honey Mustard

MAKES 4 SERVINGS

CHICKEN

Coconut oil or ghee (clarified butter)

$1^1/_2$ cups almond flour

$^1/_4$ cup arrowroot powder

$^1/_2$ cup unsweetened shredded coconut

2 teaspoons garlic powder

2 teaspoons paprika

1 teaspoon garlic salt

2 large eggs

4 boneless, skinless chicken thighs or legs

DIPPING SAUCE

$^1/_4$ cup Dijon mustard

2 tablespoons honey

Preheat the oven to 400°F. Line a baking sheet with parchment paper and brush the paper with coconut oil or ghee.

Make the chicken: In a shallow bowl, combine the almond flour, arrowroot powder, coconut, garlic powder, paprika, and garlic salt. Mix well.

In another shallow bowl, whisk the eggs.

Dip each chicken piece in the egg wash, then coat evenly with the flour mixture. Place on the baking sheet. Bake for 14 to 20 minutes, turning once, until an instant-read thermometer inserted in the thickest portion registers 165°F and the juices run clear.

Meanwhile, make the dipping sauce: In a small bowl, blend together the mustard and honey. When chicken is done, serve with the dipping sauce.

Step 7. Drink 1 Tablespoon Apple Cider Vinegar (Diluted in 3 Tablespoons Water) or Lemon Tea Daily

Yes, there is method to this madness. Apple cider vinegar, fresh ginger, and lemon all help to correct your pH, shifting you to a more alkaline state while stimulating the production of bile. This helps the gallbladder and liver break fats down effectively, lowering your blood sugar and insulin levels. In fact, some studies show that apple cider vinegar and water actually reverse NAFLD (non-alcoholic fatty liver disease), which is common to women in perimenopause or menopause, and in all women with insulin resistance and obesity. These drinks also influence the microbiome, the sea of healthy bacteria in your gut, reducing inflammation and having a positive effect on cravings for sugar, salt, and refined foods.

Note: You should never drink any vinegar without diluting it, as it can burn the back of your throat. That's why the instruction here to dilute it in water. An alternative I like is to add just a pinch of honey to my Ginger-Lemon Tea for a bit of sweetness.

Ginger-Lemon Tea
MAKES 1 SERVING
$3/4$ cup water
1 teaspoon grated fresh ginger
$1/2$ lemon, cut in half and squeezed for its juice
1 teaspoon honey

Place the water and ginger into a small saucepan and bring to a boil. Pour into a mug and add the lemon juice and honey. Stir and sip.

Note: I sometimes mix up a batch of grated ginger and lemon juice, place it in a jar, and store in the fridge. That way I can take it out and just add boiling water and honey. It's yummy both ways.

Step 8. Have 1 to 2 Teaspoons of MCT Oil Daily

MCT oil, or medium-chain triglycerides, helps hormone balance by strengthening the gut–hormone connection. This often neglected healthy fat is a medium-chain fatty acid that balances the gut microbiome, which you know now is the good bacteria in the gut. It's hard to get medium- and short-chain fatty acids through diet; in fact, this common deficiency is linked to inflammation, *Candida* overgrowth, and weight gain. The MCT oils are easier on the digestive system than fat in meats, dairy, or butter; are processed in the liver and lymph glands; and are supportive of the distribution and elimination of toxins. Consider adding MCT oil to your salads or drizzling it on top of your favorite veggies.

Sources of MCT Oil	Daily Goals
Avocado oil	$\frac{1}{4}$-$\frac{1}{2}$ teaspoon
Coconut oil	$\frac{1}{2}$ teaspoon
Ghee (clarified butter)	$\frac{1}{4}$ teaspoon
Olive oil	1 tablespoon

Step 9. Add Gut-Friendly Supplements

As you continue building a healthy gut, you'll find that gut-healthy supplements are your next natural step. Healing a leaky gut, balancing the microbiome, and improving digestion all form the foundation for optimal gut-liver-hormone balances. So, let's take a look at three kinds of gut-healthy supplements.

Probiotics

There's debate about the benefits of probiotics, but a high-quality, multi-strain probiotic has helped so many of my patients, and research continues to support the role of probiotics in overall gut health and hormone metabolism. Remember the estrabolome? Or the gut-thyroid connection? Those were discussed in Part I of this book. I prefer a product that has at least 50 billion CFU (colony-forming units) and is clearly labeled with four or five microbial strains. There is some decrease in the viability of a probiotic over time, so picking higher strains that have been well tested is key to having a product that works for you. Ideally, the probiotic should contain a mix of *Lactobacillus*, *Bifidobacterium* and *Saccharomyces boulardii*.

Digestive enzymes

Digestive enzymes, including amylase, lipase, and protease, assist in breaking foods down and delivering them to where they need to go. The body starts producing fewer digestive enzymes over time as the gut gets more sluggish, leading to bloating, constipation, reflux, and additional symptoms. This further aggravates the gut–hormone foundation, leading to hormone conditions that include estrogen dominance, low progesterone, and high insulin level.

I have so many patient stories, but I clearly remember one in which my patient started taking digestive enzymes and miraculously lost the weight in a few weeks that she had been struggling to lose for a long time. Now—fair warning!—her experience may not replicate repeatedly, but it does illustrate that these enzymes are an important piece of the hormone puzzle.

Glutamine

Glutamine is an amino acid that rebuilds the gut lining and is one of my favorite supplements for healing a leaky gut. This powerful amino acid has many other functions as well, including helping with muscle recovery, immune function, and even athletic function. Leaky gut, as we have discussed, prevents the nutrient absorption that is critical for hormone balance. Glutamine is one of the most effective ways to reverse a leaky gut and reestablish a healthy gut lining.

I recommend 1 gram of glutamine daily, added to water, juice, or your favorite smoothie. I prefer the powder form of glutamine, especially for a digestive system that may already be weak.

Customizing It—Finding Your Hormone Pattern

You've been building a solid foundation, for sure. Now, as you enter the third week of the Thirty-Day Hormone Reset, it's time for a more tailored approach. You will identify your dominant hormone pattern to receive some recommendations specific to your body and, at the same time, build on the last two weeks.

Step 10. Take the Hormone Quiz

This is the time to diverge a bit and customize your plan based on your hormone pattern, or the dominant hormone that is primarily responsible for your symptoms of Hormone Hell. All the hormones, as you have learned, do indeed work together, but there usually is a prime driver responsible for the chaos you feel. Now, you are going to identify that key influencer by taking a simple quiz that your lab results will often support. There is an abundance of information on hormones, as you have already seen, but focusing and prioritizing on the main character (as my daughter calls it) is what ultimately yields results.

As you take the quiz that follows, you will discover the primary Hormone Hell–raiser your plan will then address. Note: One assumption I am going to be so bold as to make is that all of us are in some state of cortisol dysfunction or adrenal fatigue; it's an epidemic, after all. So, whether you are a Rock Star, Hustler, Superstar, Superwoman, or Commander, the undercurrent of cortisol dysregulation is more than likely a reality. Therefore, all hormone plans assume you are in some state of adrenal fatigue and cortisol dysfunction—that's the reality of what I see every day in practice.

	A	B	C
1. I break out with acne on my chin, jaw, or neck. Y N. If yes to one or more, check column A.			
2. I often get palpitations or feel anxious at random times throughout the month. Y N. If yes, check column B.			
3. I tend to store weight around my midsection, on my arms, or on my back. Y N. If yes, check column C.			
4. I get migraine headaches, have breast tenderness, or feel bloated. Y N. If yes, check column A.			
5. My cycles are getting shorter and more frequent, or heavier, or I just don't get a cycle. Y N. If yes, check column B.			
6. I feel fatigued after eating carbohydrates and/or have high cholesterol and blood sugar levels. Y N. If yes, check column C.			
7. I have fibroids, ovarian cysts, or endometriosis, or I am post-hysterectomy for these issues. Y N. If yes, check column A.			
8. I have cravings for sugar and salt, feel cold frequently, and/or have thinning eyebrows or eyelashes. Y N. If yes, check column B.			
9. Regardless of how much I exercise or cut my carbs and sugar, it's hard for me to lose inches or pounds. Y N. If yes, check column C.			
10. I have thinning hair at the top of my scalp or at the temples, with the texture of my hair changing as well. Y N. If yes, check column A.			
Total			

Count the number of times you checked columns A, B, or C. Then circle the hormone pattern and note the most common pattern that appears:

Mostly A column: Type 1

Mostly B column: Type 2

Mostly C column: Type 3

Dominant Patterns

Did you find there's a dominant pattern for you? I hope so! If you need a backup for your conclusion, use the lists of hormone tests (see page 124) to check your levels and confirm your suspicions.

Now, let's get to customizing the plan. Based on your dominant pattern, choose your plan from the following:

Type 1: Estrogen/Androgen Dominance (follows)

Type 2: Low Progesterone/Thyroid Imbalance (see page 303)

Type 3: Insulin Resistance (see page 307)

Type 1—Estrogen/Androgen Dominance

This 16th day, you continue steps 1 through 9 of the foundational plan and add a few more to-do's to help break up and better metabolize the estrogens and androgens. Remember, androgens are also produced when testosterone or estrogen levels get too high, causing the symptoms of acne, hair loss, bloating, fibroids, migraines, and breast tenderness. Both poorly metabolized estrogen or estrogen dominance, as well as high androgens, cause mood disorders, including anxiety, depression, and general fatigue.

For your next steps, it's time to expand the options, but only after you complete the Hormone Quiz in step 10 (see page 298).

Step 11. Hormone Metabolizers: Add Four Additional Servings of Cruciferous Vegetables Weekly

One of the critical Eastern medicine ideas around hormones is the importance of hormone metabolism, or not just making hormones but how they are processed through the body. Cruciferous vegetables contain indole-3-carbinol and insoluble fiber, which helps to metabolize estrogen. Add these veggies to your favorite stir-fries or steam them for more crunch. I love coating the veggies with a little olive oil, salt, and garlic pepper, then roasting them in the air fryer. This is my go-to swap when I am craving chips, popcorn, or salty snacks.

Cruciferous vegetable include the following:

Broccoli
Brussels sprouts
Cauliflower
Leafy greens, including arugula, collard greens, dandelion greens,
    kale, mustard greens
Radishes
Rutabaga
Turnips
Watercress

Reminder: One serving is a $\frac{1}{2}$ cup of the items listed above.

Tip: Cut up all the veggies and store them in ziplock bags or glass containers so they're ready to stir-fry, air-fry, or roast whenever needed.

Step 12. Add 1 Tablespoon Cold-Pressed Organic Olive Oil Daily

Not only does olive oil have omega-6, it also has omega-9 fats, which help metabolize estrogen. Each day, add 1 tablespoon of unheated olive oil to your favorite dishes, toasts, or low-heat recipes, since olive oil has a low smoke point. (Bonus: Olive oil is great for your hair and skin, too.)

Step 13. Consider Changing to the Hormone-Metabolizing Supplements DIM, Calcium D-glucarate, or Saw Palmetto

On days 1 through 14 of your next cycle if you are menstruating, or three days per week if your cycles are irregular, or you are in menopause or have amenorrhea, we will be adding one of the following supplements known to help with metabolizing estrogen and androgens. Note: Please only add one, not all three:

DIM (diindolylmethane) if your symptoms are specific to breast tenderness, migraines, heavy bleeding, or bloating
Calcium D-glucarate if you are unsure
Saw palmetto (400 mg) if your symptoms are consistent with acne or hair loss

Step 14. Add 1 Tablespoon of Psyllium Husk or Flax Seed Daily

Psyllium husk and flax seed (ground flax seeds) are fiber sources that help better metabolize both estrogens and androgens. Consider mixing them in water or juice, or adding the flax seed to your favorite smoothies; don't add the psyllium husk to your smoothies as it will expand in liquid. Personal experience speaking here.

> ### Tips for Exercise
>
> Estrogen and androgen dominance often coexist with insulin resistance, the Type 3 hormone pattern we have identified. Keeping this in mind, exercise and movement are important parts of your hormone reset. Aim to move in twenty-minute bursts two or three times a day, adding moderate cardio and light weights to help with estrogen and androgen metabolism. Extreme exercise regimens, however, add stress and can increase androgen levels, so tracking your heart rate and keeping it to no more than 20 to 30 beats above your resting heart rate is a reasonable goal for your hormone reset.

Turn to page 312 to continue with the Thirty-Day Hormone Reset, or read on below to learn about Type 2 and Type 3 protocols.

Type 2—Low Progesterone/Thyroid Imbalance

If the hormone quiz identified dominant hormone drivers and you landed here, then you, like many women, live with the symptoms of low progesterone: anxiety, heart palpitations, sugar and salt cravings, shorter or irregular period cycles, and heavy cycles. But your thyroid may be involved as well, contributing to these symptoms but adding a few more: feeling cold and thinning hair (eyebrows and eyelashes included). Studies show that low progesterone and low thyroid hormones are related, and as progesterone levels increase, the thyroid hormone levels improve as well.

Step 11. Hormone Boosters: Add Progesterone and Thyroid-Boosting Foods

Foods high in magnesium, zinc, and iodine help boost levels of progesterone and thyroid hormones. Consider adding five servings per week of the following:

Nuts (almonds, Brazil nuts, walnuts, cashews)

Mix them up or have them straight, but watch the serving size. The goal is to eat seven to ten nuts a day at most, as a way to help increase zinc and magnesium for healthy progesterone and thyroid balance. Brazil nuts are high in selenium as well, but you need only two or three of them to get your daily selenium dose.

Pumpkin seeds

High in magnesium and zinc, pumpkin seeds are hormone superboosters, improving progesterone and thyroid levels. Aim for no more than 1 to 2 tablespoons a day.

Eggs and poultry

Eggs and poultry have lots of magnesium, zinc, and protein to help boost progesterone and thyroid levels. Aim for three or four servings per week.

Many of the recipes we have listed include eggs, nuts, and seeds. You can be creative with adding these into any of the recipes or just having fun on your own.

Step 12. Add Chaste Tree Berry Powder and Evening Primrose Oil Daily

Chaste tree berries stimulate progesterone and have been used in Eastern and herbal medicine for thousands of years. Sometimes this herb can also increase estrogen levels, so monitoring is key. The standard dose for the powder is 500 milligrams per day. Evening primrose oil contains GLA (gamma linolenic acid), an essential fatty acid that boosts progesterone levels as well. For this, I recommend 1 gram a day to help women with low progesterone.

Step 13. Mineral Balance for Hormones

Minerals play an important role in hormone boosting. Zinc, for example, is needed for testosterone, magnesium for hormone pathways and sleep, and calcium for estrogen metabolism. While some of you may have started magnesium in step 5 to help with sleep, magnesium may need more attention. Magnesium really is a miracle mineral, more powerful than its counterparts. Regulating hundreds of biochemical processes in the body, magnesium is fundamental for proper thyroid and progesterone balance. While magnesium-rich foods are a part of the reset (nuts, seeds, leafy greens), adding a magnesium supplement that is chelated with multiple forms of magnesium promotes healthy progesterone and thyroid levels. I like starting with 200 milligrams of a chelated magnesium and going either up or down in dosing from there, depending on side effects. The ideal dose is around 400 milligrams a day, but some people experience stomach cramping and diarrhea at this dose and may need smaller amounts—sometime even as low as 50 milligrams. If you already started this in Phase 1 to help your sleep, you are one step ahead.

Step 14. To Do or Not to Do: Hormone Replacement Therapy

This is the step that starts to move into the world of hormone replacement therapy (HRT). I get so many questions about HRT—what I think of it and whether it the right thing to do. Here is my answer: micro-dosing bio-identical hormones is beneficial for patients not responding to the gut-liver, food, and supplement/herbal approach.

Many of my patients who are extensively depleted need progesterone or thyroid replacement; again, they don't have the *qi* or bandwidth to build hormones naturally. For these patients, I often start bio-identical progesterone at 15 milligrams on days 16 through 28 of the cycle for menstruating women, or three days per week for women who are more irregular or not getting their periods owing to perimenopause or menopause; we then often move up from there. I prefer creams or vaginal suppositories over pills, but again, these decisions are based on the individual.

Thyroid hormones should also be adjusted to fit the patient, and this is an area that needs lots of provider support. Each patient benefits from a particular type of thyroid hormone, as discussed in Chapter 3, but my preference is for bio-identical thyroid hormones like NP Thyroid or Nature Thyroid, or a combination of Tirosint and Cytomel (gluten-free T4 and T3).

Often this hormone pattern is a depletion state, or what is called yin-deficient state in Chinese medicine. Extreme exercise, marathons, high-intensity interval training (HIIT) or classes, and using heavy weights are often not advised or should be limited. A more balanced exercise program—one that alternates gentle cardio, medium weights, and adrenaline-lowering exercises like yoga and Pilates—is often best. But still—remember to move everyday!

Turn to page 312 to continue with the Thirty-Day Hormone Reset, or read on to learn about the third dominant type.

Type 3—Insulin Resistance

It's an epidemic. Stubborn insulin levels, elevated glucose numbers, belly fat, visceral fat, liver fat—fat that just won't move. Women come to me daily, depressed about their weight, especially their amount of body fat, and they are tired of trying everything and anything to lose weight, only to be disappointed again.

What is happening here? Why the lack of movement?

It all connects to the central concept of insulin resistance, or the body's impaired response to insulin, which results in ever higher levels of glucose floating around in the body, forcing the pancreas to release more insulin, leading to more fat storage. Tricking the body to get out of this situation is, well, tricky. The body is in a comfort zone; it does not want to change. This state, or Kapha dosha in Ayurvedic medicine, results in a slow and sluggish metabolism; it needs a jump-start.

If your quiz result showed you as Type 3, your insulin and blood sugar levels might need help and are likely causing you to store fat. Continue with steps 1 to 10 for the first two weeks of your plan, and then move on to your customized plan, as follows.

Step 11. Cycle Fasting and Insulin Resistance

Yes, we are going there! If you landed here with insulin resistance as your dominant hormone pattern, then cycle fasting is right for you—not just the twelve-hour overnight fast that everyone benefits from, but also one that is slightly longer, up to sixteen hours. Here is the catch: this longer fast should be done only two days per week.

This pattern means that two days per week you eat from 12 p.m. to 8 p.m., followed by sixteen hours of fasting, or gut rest. But this does not mean you can eat whatever you like during that eight-hour eating window. Instead, you eat to accomplish the following macro amounts:

Macro Goals

- Protein: 80 grams
- Fat: 30–40 grams
- Sugar: Under 25 grams
- Carbs: Under 200 grams
- Salt: Under 1,500 mg
- Fiber: 40 grams per day

Each of these macros works to assist in lowering the insulin resistance, making the body more efficient at processing sugar and regulating insulin. Fasting and gut rest have been shown to lower lipids and Hgb A1C (blood sugar markers) and reduce visceral fat—as long as it not done for an extended period of time.

This magical macro formula can usually help you get the calories right, but it requires you to be strategic in your food planning. I hate tracking, by the way—talk about feeling deprived and negative—but smartphone apps like My Fitness Pal can make it easier. You don't have to do it forever, just a few weeks is usually enough time to get the hang of healthy portion size, nutrient quality, and nutrient need.

Step 12. Add Foods that Beat Insulin Resistance

The foods that will beat insulin resistance are those you have seen peppered through this book—all foods with specific nutritional value but also contributing to control of blood sugar levels in the body, which is, as you know, the ultimate source of inflammation and chronic disease.

ing for signs of blood sugar dips, including getting lightheaded or dizzy. If this does happen, dial back on the dose and focus more on the super-powered foods. Start with one of the two herb blends listed below for better blood sugar control.

Berberine

This chemical found in some plants like European barberry and goldenseal acts almost like a natural metformin (a drug used to treat Type 2 diabetes), reducing insulin levels and stabilizing the blood sugar. I like using this supplement in six-week bursts, as prolonged use can impact the liver. The standard dose is 500 milligrams to start, increasing to 1 gram per day.

Gymnema

This is an Ayurvedic herb (*Gymnema sylvestre*) that helps to regulate blood sugar as well. The standard dose is 400 milligrams per day.

Step 14. Decision Time: Medications, Peptides, and Shots

Oh, my!

Like hormone replacement therapy, there are times when foods, supplements, and exercise are simply not enough. For truly stubborn insulin resistance, we in practice at CentreSpringMD sometimes use metformin (an insulin-regulating prescription pharmaceutical) or other weight control therapies depending on what is appropriate for the individual patient. All these need supervision by a medical team and should only be introduced after you have followed the hormone reset system for two to three weeks. We have seen insulin resistance return if the work of building *qi*, cleaning the liver and gut, and reducing inflammation was not addressed.

In fact, beating insulin resistance is really all about adopting an anti inflammatory, Mediterranean-style diet.

You have already gotten rid of the non-nutritious foods (see pag 266), but now you are bringing the following foods into your diet fo times a week to continue to see that insulin resistance disappear:

Beans	Nuts
Eggs	Seeds
Fatty fishes (mackerel,	Vegetables
salmon, tuna)	Water (surprise, right! Yes,
Fresh fruits	this equals 8 cups a day
Leafy greens	Whole grains
Lentils	

This is your week to work on healthy swaps that help to beat in resistance. Replace a traditional sandwich with a leafy green and fish. Increase your water intake. Ditch the sugar for fresh fruit. to bring these foods into your daily routine and you will natura longer want all the junk and processed foods that make insulin tance worse.

Step 13. Supplements and Herbs to Beat Insulin Resistance

By now you know that my preference is to go natural, first startir food choices, and then adding a few supplements and herbs th good track records for bringing insulin levels down. Many of t plements introduced in the gut–liver cleanup (Chapter 6) als insulin resistance, so you have already been working on this in during the last two weeks.

Both of the following herbs should be started slowly, whil

Exercise for Type 3 Women

Exercise for treating this hormone pattern needs to be daily, vigorous, and challenging. Insulin responds to more weight training, as well as cardio, when you are doubling your heart rate—but of course, if you are depleted, this goal is not realistic. This is exactly why the first few weeks of the hormone reset are spent building *qi* to power you on the Journey UP.

Add Muscle with Weight Training—for ALL Women

I meet so many women who tell me that they walk at least a couple of miles every day, or do other aerobic exercise or yoga regularly. That's wonderful to hear, as exercise is not only fantastic and much-needed for cardiovascular health and overall well-being but also is one of the most stress-relieving activities you can do. I love yoga and do it all the time. And while cardio is great, as we get older it's especially important that we add weight-bearing exercise to our routines because it strengthens our bones.

If you're really trying to beat the metabolic clock that ticks slower with age, you've got to *weight train*. Muscle building is absolutely key. You might be wondering what bone strength and muscle building have to do with hormone health, but muscle tissue is more metabolically active than any other tissue. That helps to keep insulin resistance down, which in turn helps to keep weight down.

And you don't need to do a lot of exercise, either. According to a study published in the *British Journal of Sports Medicine* in February 2022, a mere thirty to sixty minutes of muscle-strengthening activity every week has been linked to a 10 to 20 percent lower risk of death from all causes, including heart disease and cancer.

If at all possible, schedule a session or two with a personal trainer, who can set you up with a weight-training routine that best suits your current fitness level. I often see women using weights at the gym but doing it all wrong, so they're not only not getting good results but could also get injured. There are also countless training videos on YouTube that you can follow, once you know the basics.

Days 24–30

Beating Adrenal Fatigue and Cortisol Dysfunction: The Mind-Body Toolbox

I started the Thirty-Day Hormone Reset with the warning that most of us have some level of cortisol dysfunction and adrenal fatigue. We may be in the early stages, when we feel chronically stressed, or we might be in the latter stages, when there is full-out "wired and tired" mode—up all night and tired all day. Now that we have built energy, cleaned out the liver and gut, reduced inflammation, and made healthy swaps, I hope you are in a better place to focus and manage your emotional and energetic body.

If you want to check back in with yourself, refer back to our emotional ladder on page 145. Have you moved up an emotional level at all? Let's check in with your energetic body, too. Where are you now holding stress, fear, anxiety—are there any remaining blockages at all? Refer to page 163 to help identify which chakra or energy block may still be of issue.

Combine this information with the numbers you have been tracking for the last few weeks. Many of these numbers can clue you into whether you are in a stress cycle and, if so, where you are within that cycle. Fast heart rate, high blood pressure, and low heart rate variability are all physical signs that you are in *adrenal fatigue*. Your body is telling you that something is off—emotionally and energetically.

This then leads to more profound disturbances in your mental body. Anxiety, depression, OCD, and ADHD are the mental signs of cortisol dysfunction, and emotional and energetic stress, and your labs (see page 124) confirm that diagnosis.

While all that cortisol is going in different directions, your emotional and mental state only worsens—in fact, maybe stop for a second to relook at your face, tongue, and pulse. There is a scheduled, well-thought-out plan that can lower those cortisol levels, repair your body, and help shift you into a more healing, calmer emotional state. Nothing improves when the body is chronically stressed, and every factor we have talked about—your gut, liver, sleep, food cravings, and hormones—are impacted by how you feel, with stress and cortisol dysregulation sabotaging your progress.

Step 15. The Five Body Alignment: Add Your Favorite Cortisol Balancers

We have spent a lot of time working on chemistry, the physicality of your nutrients, gut, liver, hormones, inflammation, sleep, exercise, and so much more. This last step is about moving your emotional and energetic states higher (and remember: progress, not perfection) to bring it all together.

To help rewire your emotional responses and get your cortisol under control, you will choose one tool that most resonates with you to use twenty minutes per day, and one or two tools you can do one to two hours per week—doctor's orders! No squirming or thinking about everyone and everything else allowed. Here's how to get started.

Strategies for Mitigating Stress

As I've gotten older, I've added many more ideas to my stress-busting toolbox. But I've found that the hardest part for most women is to actually set aside the time to *do* them. It's crucial for us to acknowledge our own needs—they are important. Everyone's response to the mind-body toolbox is different, but your job during this last week of the hormone reset is to find a cortisol-balancing strategy that works for YOU. This is a critical part of the Journey UP.

If you normally turn to exercise for stress relief, that's great. But this step of the plan is *in addition* to whatever exercise regimen you already follow. While some forms of exercise balance stress, others increase it and make cortisol dysregulation worse. That's where the cortisol balancers come into play.

The 20-Minute Emotional Reset

The majority of women I meet are already pulled in multiple directions throughout the day, so twenty minutes in the morning is often the most doable, realistic, and opportune time to reset your nervous system. That means no checking your emails or social media right after you wake up in the morning, Instead, set aside this early time of the day to connect to your energy center, to breathe from your diaphragm, and to center your thoughts.

I personally love meditation in the morning, and I often alternate between apps that help me (Headspace, Calm) and sound baths on Spotify. Given my innate restlessness, I may flip and journal instead, and this is also my time for prayer and connection to my spirit. But that's me—what about you?

Breathwork

Our failure to breathe in all the way down to our diaphragms, expanding our belly and extending air down into our pelvis, is one of the primary drivers of cortisol dysfunction. Shallow or surface breathing increases the blood pressure and heart rate, triggers anxiety, and can ultimately lead to pelvic floor dysfunction. So, be sure to breathe like a baby does, expanding your stomach when breathing rather than raising your shoulders.

There are many different types of breathwork that you can try; just pick one and focus.

4:7:8 Breath

Controlled breathing with counts of 4, 7, and 8 is based on an ancient yogic technique called pranayama, *and it's often done during yoga sessions. Here's how to do it:*

1. Close your lips and inhale silently through your nose for a count of 4.
2. Hold that breath for a count of 7.
3. Exhale slowly through your mouth, making a whooshing sound, for a count of 8.

Box Breathing

This is a simple breathing technique whereby you breathe in counts of 4.

1. Breathe in for a count of 4.
2. Hold for a count of 4.
3. Breathe out slowly for a count of 4.
4. Hold for a count of 4. Then start over.

Pursed Lip Breathing

This type of breathing involves breathing in and out through pursed, slightly parted lips.

Breathe in for 2 counts and out for 4 counts.

Alternate Nostril Breathing

Breathing in through the nose while closing one nostril, then through the alternate nostril, helps to regulate breath and slow us down.

Mindfulness Journaling

I have been inspired to journal ever since reading Julia Cameron's book *The Artist's Way.* That process and methodology of journaling on blank pages every morning sets the tone for my day, and I believe it has ultimately changed my life.

It's a bit like taking out the garbage and fitting a clean bag into your trash can. You are starting fresh, decluttering your busy mind and helping move yourself forward to the day at hand. Journaling can provide clarity and force you to have empathy for yourself.

For me, the mornings work best for journaling, as it sets my intentions for the day. I write down what I hope to accomplish or what might be bothering me. Alternatively, you might find it helpful to write at night before bed, looking back on the day's accomplishments (or its frustrations). Either way, journaling regularly is both calming and productive.

If you have children and you journal at night when they're still awake, make it clear to them that Mommy is not to be disturbed during this time. And suggest that they keep their own journals, or write stories, or read books during your quiet time.

Guided Meditations

If you find it hard to meditate, guided meditations can be helpful, especially those of us with busy brains or heavy hearts. Having to focus on someone else who is talking can calm you down and allow you to concentrate on what's being said. There are many apps and guided meditation resources available online; some are free while others have a small charge. Check out the following:

Buddhify

Calm

Headspace: Meditations and Sleep

Healthy Minds Program

Insight Timer

Live Awake podcast

Meditation Minis podcast

Meditation Oasis podcast

Simple Habit

Unplug

The Walk

Walking is a form of meditation. While you are surrounding yourself in nature, and getting time with your thoughts, a twenty-minute walk at any time will help lower cortisol and blood pressure, improving your overall hormone profile. This walk should be *movement*, not exercise; the activity is for your mind and spirit, not a calorie-burning one.

Mazes, walking circles, and forest bathing are all forms of meditative walk. And if you have a computer desk job, this may be your favorite twenty minutes of the whole day.

Yoga

Yoga is my favorite stress-busting technique. I have a whole toolbox of stress-busters—acupuncture, massage, mindfulness journaling, seeing my friends (I couldn't live without them!), and the others—but yoga will always be my favorite. The beauty of yoga is that it can be as long or as short, as intense or as relaxing as you want it to be. You may be a yin yogi, or more into power flow, but through it all your breath becomes united with your movement, releasing stored emotions, stress, and anxiety.

A few yoga stretches can count toward your twenty minutes of cortisol-busting, or you can try a longer routine. Following are some of my favorite poses if you want to start now with this cortisol balancer:

Child's Pose
Corpse Pose
Downward Dog
Happy Baby Pose
Mountain Pose
Prayer Pose
Seated Forward Bend
Seated Twist
Tree Pose

Take seven to ten breaths in each of these poses for three to five cycles in the morning. It's a game changer!

Weekly Energy Rewiring

In addition to the twenty-minute emotional reset, we need a one- to two-hour weekly relaxer. Energetic rewiring is the time-out period you set strictly for yourself. I don't know about you, but I look forward to this special time—and when I don't get it, I definitely feel off my game. You choose your time-out period to suit yourself, but here is a list of cortisol-balancing activities that you might add to your calendar, something essential for your to-do list. Any of these can fill your two-hour self-care weekly time slot, whether you do them for two hours straight or split them to fit smaller time slots:

Acupuncture
Ayurvedic treatments—shriodhara, abhygangha

Biking (not spinning)
Craniosacral therapy
Energy healing
Golf
Hiking
Massage
Reiki
Swimming
Yoga

You could probably add to this list, but pick something you love doing and roll with it—your hormones will thank you.

What follows is an outline of the plan you can use for quick reference to help you stay on track throughout the journey:

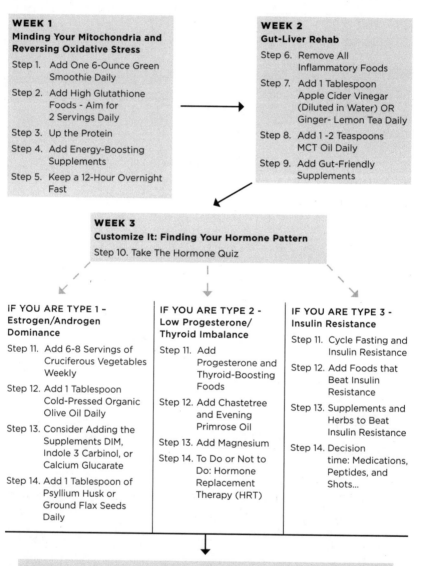

WEEK 1
Minding Your Mitochondria and Reversing Oxidative Stress

Step 1. Add One 6-Ounce Green Smoothie Daily

Step 2. Add High Glutathione Foods - Aim for 2 Servings Daily

Step 3. Up the Protein

Step 4. Add Energy-Boosting Supplements

Step 5. Keep a 12-Hour Overnight Fast

WEEK 2
Gut-Liver Rehab

Step 6. Remove All Inflammatory Foods

Step 7. Add 1 Tablespoon Apple Cider Vinegar (Diluted in Water) OR Ginger- Lemon Tea Daily

Step 8. Add 1-2 Teaspoons MCT Oil Daily

Step 9. Add Gut-Friendly Supplements

WEEK 3
Customize It: Finding Your Hormone Pattern

Step 10. Take The Hormone Quiz

IF YOU ARE TYPE 1 – Estrogen/Androgen Dominance

Step 11. Add 6-8 Servings of Cruciferous Vegetables Weekly

Step 12. Add 1 Tablespoon Cold-Pressed Organic Olive Oil Daily

Step 13. Consider Adding the Supplements DIM, Indole 3 Carbinol, or Calcium Glucarate

Step 14. Add 1 Tablespoon of Psyllium Husk or Ground Flax Seeds Daily

IF YOU ARE TYPE 2 - Low Progesterone/ Thyroid Imbalance

Step 11. Add Progesterone and Thyroid-Boosting Foods

Step 12. Add Chastetree and Evening Primrose Oil

Step 13. Add Magnesium

Step 14. To Do or Not to Do: Hormone Replacement Therapy (HRT)

IF YOU ARE TYPE 3 - Insulin Resistance

Step 11. Cycle Fasting and Insulin Resistance

Step 12. Add Foods that Beat Insulin Resistance

Step 13. Supplements and Herbs to Beat Insulin Resistance

Step 14. Decision time: Medications, Peptides, and Shots...

WEEK 4
Beating Adrenal Fatigue and Cortisol Dysfunction: The Mind-Body Toolbox

Step 15. Add Your Favorite Cortisol Balancers

And that concludes the Thirty-Day Hormone Reset. How are you? How do you feel? Where are your numbers now? Where are you on the emotional spectrum? Take a few minutes to observe and write down the following numbers:

My Vital Signs

My Numbers

  RHR:

  HRV:

  BP:

  BBT:

Dominant emotion:

Tongue:

Face:

Energy center:

Do you feel more hopeful and alive, or at least that things are moving in the right direction? The journey to hormone balance continues past these thirty days. But this is your basic plan, with its identification of your dominant hormone pattern, your biorhythm, rehab of your gut-liver connection, and restructuring of your habits. This plan has introduced you to the herbs and supplements that can heal, as well as the mind-body tools necessary to live our superpowered lives. This is the beginning of aligning your five bodies.

From here on, you may find you need more hormone support, possibly in the form of hormone replacement therapy, other medications, or even more diagnostic imaging. (Check out my rescuer remedy guide in the Resources on page 327.) With the right medical team in place, you can navigate those decisions from the vantage point of having constructed a healthy hormone foundation and having gained a deeper understanding of how your hormones work, what to look for, and when to act.

Your next move is to wait—wait to claim your energy and power with a sense of abundance and strength. You wait to *give* yourself that standing ovation that will celebrate how you finally got here, you journeyed through these pages, you took a deeper look at yourself, and you fed your cells while balancing your hormones. You are ready for anything now, having moved from the fear and instability of the first and second chakra, up to wisdom, intuition, and expression of your deepest desires—your fourth, fifth, and sixth chakras.

You have dumped the baggage, cleared the blockages, and balanced your chemistry. Your cells and your soul are in alignment, your five bodies merging. Now—go forth and conquer!

epilogue

The Journey UP

I hate endings. But this ending can be a new beginning for you. You have combed through the pages and completed the thirty days of the hormone reset. You are, more than likely, already seeing hormonal shifts; they may be subtle, with a little more energy here, a brighter smile now, fewer hot flashes or night sweats, and a general feeling of greater ease and contentment. You have done the work. You have started your own Journey UP.

As you have seen, balancing your hormones leads to balance in all five of your bodies—mental, physical, emotional, energetic, and social. You have a sharper mind, better libido, greater fertility, and higher energy. Perimenopause and menopause have become manageable hormone shifts, rather than an ending to life. Adolescent hormone imbalance and PCOS have an explanation and a plan. And as you feel better, you become unstoppable. So, yes, you should begin that job, start that business, adopt that child, get married or divorced, trek the Himalayas, or swim with the dolphins. You should be doing that which you were born to do—your soul's mission in action.

I want all women to navigate hormone shifts gracefully, evolving with each one, and becoming a better and more authentic version of their younger selves. If that's you, you are finally stepping into your power, having gained the lessons of previous decades; the hits, the losses, the wins, all have guided you with sails steady in the wind. But your chemistry has to cooperate, so you have to continue to do the work. You have to take the time to understand that chemistry and prepare for changes and shifts. What does your body need now so that your brain and heart can thrive? Where is your energy? What is your mood? Are you in pain? These obstacles will block your purpose and crush your passion if you don't act. Honestly, all women, from ages thirteen to seventy, should be asking these questions. This is how we all dump the baggage.

If you start to have symptoms of a hormone shift, that's your call to action—get the help you deserve. Prepare for those hormone shifts just as you prepare for other shifts in your life. The secret to success is making sure you return to that commitment to yourself. And if you do stumble, go back to the beginning of the plan and identify the emotional and energetic blocks that may have surfaced. Give yourself grace, and remember: *it's not you, it's your hormones.*

Life has a habit of always getting in the way, but the highs and lows are there to make us all better, stronger, and wiser—or to put us on a path that is more congruent with our soul's mission. Thus, this foundational plan for hormone balance will serve you through the transitions and along the journeys we all take as women, through the good and the bad, the ups and the downs, the wins and the losses. Ultimately, our purpose is to be in motion, see our passion is action, and embrace the Journey UP.

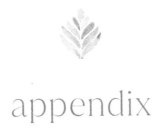

appendix

Doctor's Visit Checklist

My symptoms:

_____

_____

_____

Hormones to check:

_____

_____

_____

Requested bloodwork/exams

_____

_____

_____

Questions to ask my physician:

_____

_____

_____

_____

_____

_____

_____

_____

_____

_____

_____

_____

Exams to consider:

Blood work

Pelvic exam

Ultrasound

Breast exam

Mammogram

Colonoscopy

Thermography

Bone scan

Standard Blood Work

Hormone	Optimal Range	My Numbers	Any Notes
DHEA	100–200 μg/dl		
Estrogen-estrone (E1)	Never over 150 pg/ml		
Estrogen-estradiol (E2)	Never over 200 pg/ml (never under 50 pg/ml unless in menopause and this is goal replacement level)		
Insulin	3–5 uIU/ml		
Hgb (A1C)	5–5.5		
Progesterone	Never less than 0.5 (also replacement goal)		
Testosterone-total	20–40 ng/dl (will be low in menopause but these are hormone replacement goals)		
Testosterone-free	1–2 ng/dl		
Thyroid TSH	1–2 mIU/L		
Thyroid total T3	100–200 ng/dl		
Thyroid total T4	5–11.5 μg/dl		

Other Hormones for Potential Testing

Hormone	Optimal Range	My Numbers	Any Notes
Cortisol (AM sample)	5–25 μg/dl		
Melatonin (night dose)	40–100 pg/ml		
Androgens	15–70 ng/dl		
Growth hormone	variable but goal is 150–250 ng/ml		
ACTH	10–60 pg/ml		
Prolactin	<20 ug/ml in non-pregnant women		

For references and more resources, please visit https://doctortaz.com.

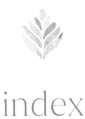

index

estrogen, 41, 88, 107–8, 141–42, 143, 222–23, 300. *see also* symptoms of hormonal imbalance
estrone, 121
exercise, 303, 306, 311, 314

fasting, 213–15, 282, 307–8
fatigue, 73–74
fat malabsorption, 186–87
fats (dietary), 188, 204–5, 208, 218, 225, 231–32
fatty liver syndrome, 236
fear, 137–38
fermented foods, 221
fiber, 217–18, 302–3
fibroids, 18, 64, 72, 78, 108, 126, 142, 165, 191, 239, 300
follicle-stimulating hormone (FSH), 113–15
food. *see* nutrition; Thirty-Day Hormone Reset
fructosamine, 121
functional Western medicine, 154–55

gallbladder, 138–39, 188–91
genetics, 39–40, 126–27, 130, 142, 200
glutamine, 194, 296–97
gluten, 208, 212–13
goiters, 88
gonadotropin-releasing hormone, 115
grief, 138–39
growth hormone, 114–15
gut-hormone connection, 177–95
  detoxification and, 250–55
  foods for support of, 221
  health issues of, 74–75, 180–91
  quiz about, 179–80
  supplements for, 192–94, 204–5
gymnema, 310

hair loss/excess hair, 4, 52, 75–76
Hashimoto's disease, 87–88
hate, 139–40
HDL (high-density lipoprotein), 188
healing modalities. *see* EastWest holistic approach
heart chakra, 135–36, 163
herbalists, 156–58
high-glutathione foods, 277–78
histamine response, 187
homeopathy, 156–58
hope, 136
hormonal imbalance, 15–145
  emotions and, 129–45, 313–19
  finding pattern, 298–300, 303, 307
  hormone dysfunction, 6
  key hormone shifts, 17–50
  symptoms of, 61–92 (*see also* symptoms of hormonal imbalance)
  understanding, 3–8, 11
Hormone Hell, 3, 21, 127. *see also* checklists; symptoms of hormonal imbalance
hormones, 93–127. *see also* dirty hormones; EastWest holistic approach; symptoms of hormonal imbalance; Thirty-Day Hormone Reset
  brain, 111–16
  circulation of, 185
  defined, 93–96
  hormone replacement therapy (HRT), 116–20, 306
  metabolism, 101–7, 240
  as root cause of emotions, 132
  sex, 107–11
  stress and sleep, 96–101
  Symptom Checklist, 62–63
  tests for, 121–27
  types of, 96–116, 240

traditional Chinese medicine
(TCM), 10, 133, 157, 168–73,
174–75, 226, 238, 256
"changes in essence," 172–73
detoxification and, 256
for diagnosis, 170–72
EastWest medicine in practice,
174–75
herbalists, 157
herbs and plants for, 226
on liver, 238
meridians, 130, 133, 135, 136, 137,
168–72, 174, 177–79, 256, 274
qi, 130, 163, 169, 190
on vitality, 10
yin-yang, 169
trans fats, 208
trauma, 6
triglycerides, 214
The 21-Day Belly Fix (Bhatia), 179,
258–59

University of Arizona, 154
uterus, 33, 71–72, 78, 299

vaginal changes, 88–89
Vatas, 159, 160, 161, 162, 165, 179
vegetables, 221
vitality, 10
vital signs, 270–72
vitamins, 198–204, 230–32

weight gain, 89–91, 186–87
weight gain/loss, 214–15

Weil, Andrew, 6
Western medicine, 150–58. *see also*
EastWest holistic approach
approach to hormone shifts,
19–22
complementary/alternative
medicine, 155
conventional, 150–53
EastWest medicine in practice,
174–75
endocrinologists, 19, 25, 52, 83,
178
functional, 154–55
gaslighting of women's health,
18–19
homeopaths, herbalists, essential
oils, 156–58
integrative medicine, 153–54
medical training, 18–19, 154,
178–79
naturopathic medicine, 155–56
understanding, 11–12
wine, 224
women's health. *see* hormones
Women's Health Initiative Study,
117
worry, 137

xenoestrogens, 244

yin-yang, 169
yoga, 317–18

zinc, 203

about the author

Tasneem Bhatia, MD, (aka Dr. Taz) is a board-certified integrative medicine physician and the founder of CentreSpringMD, an award-winning medical and wellness practice in Atlanta, Georgia. She gained national recognition as the author of the books *What Doctors Eat*, *The 21-Day Belly Fix*, and *Super Woman RX*. Her integration of Eastern medical wisdom with modern science has led to featured segments on *TODAY*, *Good Morning America*, and CNN, and eventually to the premiere of her own PBS special *Super Woman RX with Dr. Taz*. Dr. Taz is dedicated to empowering women to radically transform their lives through personalized approaches to lifestyle, diet, exercise, and self-care. As a proud member of the Southeast board for UNICEF USA, she is committed to improving the health of children and families around the world.